Men's Health

Life Improvement Guides®

Vitamin Vitality

Use Nature's Power
to Attain
Optimal Health

by Donna Raskin, Brian Paul Kaufman,
and the Editors of Men'sHealth Books

Rodale Press, Inc.
Emmaus, Pennsylvania

Other titles in the *Men's Health Life Improvement Guides* series:

Fight Fat	*Sex Secrets*
Food Smart	*Stress Blasters*
Maximum Style	*Stronger Faster*
Powerfully Fit	*Symptom Solver*

Library of Congress Cataloging-in-Publication Data

Raskin, Donna.
    Vitamin vitality : use nature's power to attain optimal health / by Donna Raskin,
Brain Paul Kaufman, and the editors of Men's Health Books.
       p.   cm.—(Men's health life improvement guides)
    Includes index.
    ISBN 0–87596–408–7 paperback
    1. Vitamins in human nutrition.   2. Minerals in human nutrition.
3. Men—Health and hygiene. I. Kaufman, Brian, 1961– . II. Men's Health Books.
III. Title. IV. Series.
QP771.R37   1997
613.2'86—dc21   97–17375

Distributed in the book trade by St. Martin's Press

2   4   6   8   10   9   7   5   3   1   paperback

—— OUR PURPOSE ——

"We inspire and enable people to improve
their lives and the world around them."

Vitamin Vitality Editorial Staff
Managing Editor: **Jack Croft**
Writers: **Donna Raskin, Brian Paul Kaufman, Brian Chichester, Margo Trott**
Assistant Research Manager: **Jane Unger Hahn**
Book Project Researcher: **Deborah Pedron**
Editorial Researchers: **Tanya H. Bartlett, Elizabeth A. Brown, Lori Davis, Jennifer L. Kaas,
Nanci Kulig, Deanna Moyer, Shea Zukowski, Alice Drake, Paris Mihely-Muchanic, Staci Ann Sander**
Copy Editors: **Linda Mooney, David R. Umla**
Series Art Directors: **Charles Beasley, Tanja L. Lipinski**
Series Designer: **John Herr**
Book Designer: **Thomas P. Aczel**
Cover Designer: **Charles Beasley**
Cover Photographer: **Mitch Mandel**
Illustrators: **Thomas P. Aczel, Alan Baseden**
Manufacturing Coordinator: **Melinda B. Rizzo**
Office Manager: **Roberta Mulliner**
Office Staff: **Julie Kehs, Mary Lou Stephen**

Rodale Health and Fitness Books
Vice-President and Editorial Director: **Debora T. Yost**
Executive Editor: **Neil Wertheimer**
Design and Production Director: **Michael Ward**
Research Manager: **Ann Gossy Yermish**
Copy Manager: **Lisa D. Andruscavage**
Studio Manager: **Stefano Carbini**
Book Manufacturing Director: **Helen Clogston**

Photo Credits
Page 152: **Courtesy Denver Broncos**
Page 154: **Courtesy NBA Photos/Philadelphia 76ers**
Page 156: **Courtesy MET–Rx**
Page 158: **Courtesy Tracy Frankel**
Back flap: **Everett Collection**

Contents

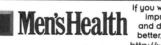

Introduction

Getting with the Program

The French philosopher E. M. Cioran once wrote: "We derive our vitality from our store of madness." Not me. I do my shopping at the store of vitamins and minerals (also known as the neighborhood pharmacy). Lately, though, I must confess that my local drugstore increasingly resembles a store of madness. The shelves are lined with all manner of pills, potions, and tablets, all boasting of incredible health benefits. And in many cases, that's literally what those boasts are: *not* credible. It has gotten to the point where it's almost impossible to tell the pills apart without a program.

Welcome to the program.

In *Vitamin Vitality*, you'll find the rock-solid information you need to separate hype from hope and medical fact from science fiction. We know that this is the information that men want because, well, they told us. As part of our ongoing efforts to make our books as useful as possible for the guys who read them, we regularly bring small groups of men together to discuss health issues that are most important to them. They often struggle—just like we do—with how to fit exercise and good eating habits into a stress-filled, jam-packed schedule. That's why we launched the *Men's Health Life Improvement Guides* in the first place.

And that's why we wrote this book in particular. When we first started thinking about what topics should be covered in this series, I'll be honest with you, vitamins weren't on the list—at least not a whole book about them. Sure, we knew that vitamins and minerals play a key role in good nutrition, but we honestly didn't think guys would be interested in an entire volume on the subject. Boy, were we wrong. And we have our readers to thank for setting us straight.

In wide-ranging, informal sessions, we talked with men from coast to coast about what specific steps they take to maintain and improve their health. And to our surprise, one after another talked about how crucial vitamin and mineral supplements are to their daily health routines. It's not that these men didn't understand the importance of eating a balanced, nutritious diet. They did. But they also were realists who understood that, despite their best intentions, it didn't always happen. And that's not all. Many also understood how vitamins and minerals could give them an edge in life against the diseases that most often kill men.

Gaining that edge is what *Vitamin Vitality* is really all about. Sure, if your main interest is maintaining good health, you'll find all of the basics covered here. We'll walk you through what you need to know about each vitamin and mineral: what it is, what role it plays in your body, and how much you need to thrive. But if you want to know how to smartly use vitamin and mineral supplements to gain that extra advantage—whether it's to ward off diseases such as cancer and heart attack, or to build muscle and boost brainpower—you'll find that here, too.

We understand the seemingly innate desire in men to get the edge. It probably dates back to prehistoric times, when being just a little bit faster or smarter than the next cave guy meant the difference between bringing home dinner and being dinner. There is, to be sure, a dark side to this primal urge. It can seduce some to turn to what are euphemistically called performance-enhancing drugs. Or to fall for the hucksterism of modern-day snake oil salesmen peddling pills that lack any scientific foundation for their wild claims.

But in nature's storehouse, you'll find what you need to live longer, stronger, and better. All you need is the key to open the door. And, as in most things in life, that key is knowledge.

Jack Croft

Jack Croft
Managing Editor, *Men's Health* Books

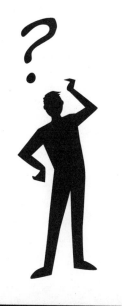

Part One

What a Man Needs

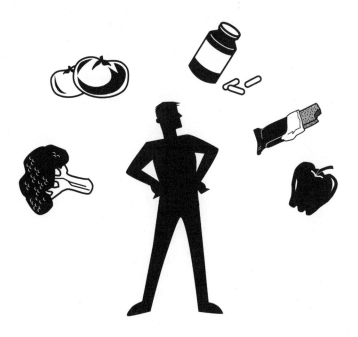

What Do You Know?

A Nutritional Self-Test

Every time you pick up the paper or turn on the news, it seems you hear about some new discovery relating to vitamins and minerals. It's tough to keep on top of all the changes.

For instance, it seems like hardly a week passes without some new study making some new claim about beta-carotene. But be honest: Do you really know what beta-carotene is? Do you know whether it is (a) a vitamin, (b) a mineral, or (c) neither? (The correct answer is neither.) Before you embark on our guided journey through the nutrient maze, take a few minutes to test your knowledge. Then, after you've completed *Vitamin Vitality*, come back and take the test again. As your score soars, so will your health—provided you put the nutritional power of your newfound knowledge into practice in your daily life.

1. **The Daily Value for vitamin C is 60 milligrams. How many milligrams did early vitamin C pioneer Linus Pauling, Ph.D., the double Nobel prize–winning doctor who wrote *Vitamin C and the Common Cold*, take every day; and how old was he when he died?**

   a. **18,000 milligrams and 62 years old**

   b. **12,000 milligrams and 93 years old**

   c. **250 milligrams and 81 years old**

   d. **1,000 milligrams and 54 years old**

2. **Which mineral joins vitamins A, C, and E as an antioxidant?**

   a. **Selenium**

   b. **Magnesium**

   c. **Iron**

   d. **Chromium**

3. **Which mineral transports oxygen in the blood?**

   a. **Chromium**

   b. **Zinc**

   c. **Sulfur**

   d. **Iron**

4. **Let's face it, you drink just a little more than your friends. This causes you to lose what?**

   a. **Sodium**

   b. **Potassium**

   c. **B vitamins, particularly thiamin**

   d. **Your balance**

5. **Why were British sailors called limeys?**

   a. **Because their faces turned the color of limes when they got seasick**

   b. **Because someone once told them to eat citrus fruits, such as limes, to combat scurvy**

   c. **Because their uniforms were lime green**

   d. **Because French sailors were called Lemonheads**

6. **You're a Caucasian man who lives in Alaska, and it's summertime. Should you take extra vitamin D or not?**

   a. **No, because your body will process vitamin D from the sun, and too much vitamin D can be dangerous.**

   b. **Yes, because there's no such thing as getting too many vitamins.**

(continued)

7. **Nuts are nutritious. They contain:**

    a. **Vitamins, particularly B_6 and B_{12}**

    b. **Protein**

    c. **Three minerals: chromium, manganese, and selenium**

8. **Folic acid, a member of the B vitamin family, has been known by many names, including:**

    a. **Popular vitamin, factor vitamin, vitamin B_3, and leaf vitamin**

    b. **Pteroylglutamic acid, Wills' factor, factor U, and vitamin M**

    c. **Vitamin B_4, skin factor H, and Preparation H**

9. **Table salt. You know it; you probably use too much of it. What two minerals are in it?**

    a. **Sodium and phosphorous**

    b. **Sodium and chloride**

    c. **Sodium and potassium**

10. **Is it okay for you to take your kid's chewable vitamin?**

    a. **No, because children's vitamins have far fewer vitamins and minerals than adult versions.**

    b. **Yes, because I probably need the same nutrients as my children.**

    c. **No, because kids' vitamins have more vitamins and minerals than adults' to help their growing bodies.**

11. **Which diseases are caused by vitamin and/or mineral deficiencies?**

    a. **Pellagra**

    b. **Beriberi**

    c. **Cretinism**

    d. **Goiter**

    e. **Night blindness**

    f. **All of the above**

12. **Which minerals have been used as money?**

    a. **Zinc and iron**

    b. **Iron and copper**

    c. **Copper and salt**

13. **What's the difference between vitamins and minerals?**

    a. **A vitamin is needed in larger amounts**

    b. **Vitamins come from organic things, minerals come from nonorganic things**

    c. **Vitamins don't have names, just letters and numbers**

    d. **All of the above**

14. **RDA is an acronym for:**

    a. **Rural Delivery Association**

    b. **Registered Dietitians Association**

    c. **Recommended Dietary Allowance**

    d. **Recommended Daily Amount**

15. **Is beta-carotene added to processed food for coloring?**

    a. **Yes, because it's a pigment that can make foods more yellow-orange.**

    b. **No, because it's found in green, leafy vegetables.**

Bonus question: Are there any vitamins or minerals in semen?

Correct answers: 1. b, 2. a, 3. d, 4. c, 5. b, 6. a, 7. c, 8. b, 9. b, 10. b, 11. f, 12. c, 13. b, 14. c, 15. a, Bonus question: Yes, vitamin C and zinc

What Are Vitamins and Minerals?

Better Living through Chemistry

In their quest to create a more tasty and attractive dish, cereal makers in the Far East began to refine rice in the mid-1800s. At the same time, a disease called beriberi, also known as polyneuritis, spread like wildfire through countries where rice made up a huge part of the average diet. The Philippine word *beriberi* translates to "I can't, I can't." Or, more descriptively, "I'm so sick I don't have the energy to get up and move around." The disease causes inflamed nerves, which leads to paralysis.

At the turn of the twentieth century, Filipino and Indonesian physicians came up with a reliable cure for beriberi, a drink called tikitiki. And what was tikitiki made from? Rice bran extract. The same part that was removed from rice during the refining process. An important connection between food and health was made. Clearly, some substance in rice bran was the key to curing beriberi. But it would be more than two decades before scientists figured out that the substance was thiamin, also known as vitamin B_1.

Of course, you can't really blame them for taking so long. When they started looking for the cure, vitamins didn't even exist.

Vital Facts

Okay, to be precise, vitamins have always been around. We just didn't have a clue what they were. That all changed in 1912, when a Polish biochemist named Casimir Funk coined the word *vitamines*. Funk believed that there was just one substance in our diets necessary for life, so he combined *vita*, Latin for "life," with *amine* because he thought that the one substance contained nitrogen. Later research showed that there were many "vitamines," but few were nitrogen-based. So the final "e" was dropped. Funk's word, however, endured. Like they used to say on *Laugh-In*, you can look *that* up in your Funk and Wagnall's.

Funk's concept also has endured. Vitamins are tiny, organic substances necessary for at least one metabolic function. In other words, necessary for life. They are essential micronutrients, which means precisely what it sounds like: very small things that your body absolutely must have for nourishment. Miss out on any of them and you risk contracting diseases. If you don't have vitamin C, you get scurvy; no vitamin A and you'll suffer from night blindness. A shortage of niacin and you'll come down with pellagra, an ugly little syndrome that leaves you with cracks and sores around your mouth; scales on the back of your hands, neck, and chest; vomiting; and diarrhea. A nutrient is a substance that you must consume because your body can't produce it.

Just because vitamins are small doesn't mean that they aren't as important as other nutrients like water, carbohydrates, fat, and protein. Vitamins act as catalysts for vital processes in the body. For example, your body converts thiamin into a coenzyme called thiamin pyrophosphate, which aids in metabolizing carbohydrates and sugars. Without thiamin, your body wouldn't be able to turn the spaghetti you eat into the energy you burn during a run.

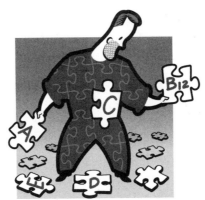

"We often think of the body as a machine analogous to a car," says Cathy Kapica, R.D., Ph.D., associate professor of nutrition and clinical dietetics at Finch University of Health Science/Chicago Medical

School. "Food with lots of nutrients is like gasoline: The higher the quality of the gasoline, the better the car runs. The same is true of your body. The higher and more varied the amount of vitamins and minerals in your food, the more likely it is that your body will run better."

Meet the Minerals

Like vitamins, some minerals are necessary for life. They are composed of various arrangements of the 92 naturally occurring elements found in the periodic table, which most of us haven't looked at since high school. Where vitamins are organic, meaning that they contain carbon atoms, minerals are nonorganic, meaning that they don't contain carbon.

Minerals come in two sizes: macronutrients and micronutrients. We need large amounts of 7 minerals, including calcium, magnesium, and potassium. But we only require trace amounts of 9 others, including zinc and iron. And there are 29 other minerals inside our bodies that scientists can't account for. Why do we need lead, mercury, and lithium? No one knows.

When it comes to minerals, size truly doesn't matter. Just because one mineral comes in trace amounts and another in huge quantities doesn't mean that the bigger one is more important. For example, calcium makes up 2 percent of a man's body weight, while iodine only represents 0.00004 percent of that same weight. But almost all of that iodine is concentrated in the thyroid gland, where it becomes part of the hormones that promote growth and regulate energy. If you don't get enough iodine, you'll develop a goiter, or enlarged thyroid gland.

While 16 minerals (both macro and micro) currently meet the "essential" criteria, researchers don't discount the importance of the

A, B, C, D, E, . . . K?

There is only one vitamin A, but there are eight B vitamins. There is a C, D, and E . . . but no F, G, or H. What's the story behind these out-of-order letters? International research and lots of backtracking.

Many scientists work on the same compounds and questions at the same time, often without knowing it. That was even more so 50 to 100 years ago, when much of the groundbreaking vitamin research was done. So, each person discovered one or more uses for a compound and then gave it a name relating to that use.

Letters were picked often just to distinguish the unstudied compounds from other more researched ones. But earning a vitamin letter is much tougher than getting a varsity letter in college. Consider poor vitamin G. Never heard of it? That's because what was originally tagged as an exciting new discovery turned out to be just another member of the B-complex brood. It now is known as riboflavin or B_2.

So how did we jump to vitamin K? It's necessary for coagulation, spelled with a "K" in Dutch, the nationality of its discoverers.

other minerals in the body. Fluoride is not considered essential, even though it's a generally accepted practice to use it as protection against tooth decay. Is it essential for life, growth, or reproduction? No. But it certainly is responsible for a lot more smiles in your life.

While scientists have, during the last two centuries, isolated the numerous vitamins and minerals in your body, they also have found that your diet, genetic history, exercise habits, age, and geographical location impact on your intake and absorption of these same vitamins and minerals, says Shari Lieberman, Ph.D., certified nutrition specialist and co-author of *The Real Vitamin and Mineral Book*.

Antioxidants and Free Radicals

The Battle for Your Body

Welcome to your bloodstream, which even as you read this, is happily transporting oxygen from the air to various sites in your body. Feels good, doesn't it? There's just one small problem. Some of that oxygen is damaged. Pollution, sunlight, cigarette smoke, and other environmental factors can damage the oxygen molecule by increasing or decreasing the number of electrons it holds. This damage can occur before you breathe the oxygen in or can occur inside your body.

An oxygen molecule wants to keep its number of electrons stable, so if one is missing or a new one appears, the molecule attempts to re-stabilize its electron supply. It will pick up an electron from a nearby molecule. That sets off a chain reaction of electron grabbing. From there it's like a pinball free-for-all inside your body. Everybody's grabbing an electron, the cells are going crazy, the radical molecules are free!

Free radicals—the name scientists came up with for these altered oxygen molecules—can cause a lot of trouble in your body. For example, they are a big contributor to the clogging of arteries. Free radicals like to steal electrons from a type of cholesterol in your blood called low-density lipoproteins, or LDLs. This damages the LDL and causes it to stick to an artery wall, which, in turn, clogs the artery.

Truth be told, some free radicals have a positive impact on your body. The immune system sometimes produces free radicals to fight infections and

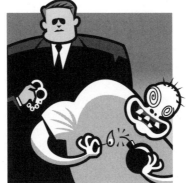

viruses, for instance. However, there is much more evidence pointing to the damage that free radicals can do than the reverse.

The best way to protect yourself against the damage done by free radicals is to discourage their replication in the first place. The experts agree: Don't smoke, try to breathe in lots of clean air, get a good amount of moderate exercise, and stay away from processed foods. And now doctors recommend that you eat—and possibly supplement your diet with—antioxidants. These include vitamins C and E and beta-carotene, the best-known of the carotenoid compounds that the body converts into vitamin A.

Meet Your Allies

When an antioxidant vitamin meets up with a free radical, it happily donates an electron to the damaged molecule. This not only restores one molecule to health but also cuts short the free-radical chain reaction. Consume enough antioxidants to counteract the oxidization process and you'll age more slowly and in better health. Think of a swing set that sits in the backyard year after year. If you covered it with a tarp during the winter, chances are that the snow wouldn't cause as much damage come next spring when it's time to play. Similarly, free radicals cause rust in your body.

According to a 1994 study done by the U.S. Department of Agriculture, many men actually consume 100 percent or more of the recommended amounts of vitamins E, C, and A. But that may not be enough to fight free radicals. "The Recommended Dietary Allowances (RDA) weren't created to combat diseases such as cancer and heart disease," says Alan Gaby, M.D., professor of therapeutic nutrition at Bastyr University in Seattle. "Now we know that antioxidants can help prevent these problems."

For example, the

Cambridge Heart Antioxidant Study (CHAOS) found that people with arteriosclerosis (blocked arteries) who took 400 to 800 international units (IU) of vitamin E had a 47 percent decrease in their risk of heart attack and death from heart attack. However, the Daily Value for vitamin E in the United States is 30 IU, a much smaller amount than the subjects in the CHAOS study took. Be advised, though, if you're considering taking more than 600 IU of vitamin E, you should first consult your doctor.

A good diet will provide you with the vitamin E that you need, says David Meyers, M.D., professor of internal medicine and preventive medicine at University of Kansas School of Medicine in Kansas City. Many people choose supplements, however, because vitamin E is found mainly in high-fat foods. "But a prudent use of olive oil and other monounsaturated fats is very reasonable," he adds.

Dr. Meyers believes supplementing with vitamin E makes sense, provided it's just part of a healthy lifestyle. "Along with eating a well-balanced diet and exercising, I take vitamin E. I figure that it's a low-risk investment that is easily affordable, so why not?"

While vitamin E's sole purpose is to act as an antioxidant, the same is not true for vitamins A and C. That's why it is important to get most of those two vitamins from food, says Dr. Meyers.

"Vitamin A comprises about 1,000 different compounds, including beta-carotene. All of these carotenoids are present in a well-balanced diet, but a beta-carotene supplement contains only one type of carotenoid," Dr. Meyers says. "How are we to know it's the most important one?"

Similarly, fruits high in vitamin C, such as oranges, contain many other healthy compounds, including fiber and bioflavonoids, which may help relieve inflammation and

Another Antioxidant Ally

Vitamins are not the only antioxidants. The mineral selenium also protects against free-radical cell damage. In fact, selenium and vitamin E, another antioxidant, work so well together that they often substitute for each other.

Selenium may also play a pivotal role in helping to prevent AIDS. In fact, studies at the University of Georgia in Athens indicate that a selenium deficiency may be the switch that turns HIV into AIDS.

Selenium seems to protect the eyes from cataracts and the heart from muscle damage, just like vitamin E. In fact, if you're deficient in vitamin E, your body may use its store of selenium to make up for the vitamin E loss, and vice versa.

allergy symptoms, among other things.

Researchers are still learning about the various ways each of the antioxidants work. Vitamin C, for example, seems to be particularly effective in fighting the damage caused by cigarettes. If you smoke and then take a vitamin C supplement, you won't "cure" the damage, but the vitamin C will lessen it. But if you quit smoking, you may not need the high doses of vitamin C anymore. In other words, vitamin C—unlike vitamin E—may not counteract free radicals in someone who already takes pretty good care of himself, Dr. Meyers says.

In fact, cautions Dr. Meyers, all the vitamins and minerals in the world can't undo the effects of smoking, a sedentary lifestyle, or bad food choices. "The effect of vitamin E is dwarfed by cigarette smoking," he says. "Vitamin E is much less powerful than daily exercise, and its effect is much smaller than achieving optimal weight and normalizing blood pressure."

In other words, no pill in the world—vitamin or not, antioxidant or not—can take the place of a healthy lifestyle.

What the Government Says You Need

Understanding RDAs and Daily Values

At the start of World War II, the Department of Defense began calling up young men to fight but found that many American guys just didn't have what it takes to go to war. Their stores of vitamins and minerals were way down, which left them with a number of deficiency diseases, such as rickets, pellagra, and anemia. To get the weakened would-be soldiers into fighting form, a number of scientists got together to form the Food and Nutrition Board of the National Research Council. The group published the first set of Recommended Dietary Allowances—immediately shortened to RDAs—in 1943. The goal was to help ensure that all citizens get the minimum amounts of nutrients necessary to stay alive and maintain satisfactory health.

And so it remains today. The RDAs are formulated to maintain good health. These are the nutrient values that are absolutely essential for healthy living.

The Food and Nutrition Board is a nongovernmental agency, but the government uses its numbers to set official labeling and dietary standards. These are the numbers and percentages you see on the back of cereal boxes and other food products.

The idea is that if you consume the levels of vitamins and minerals set by the board, you'll be protected from deficiency diseases. For example, if you get the RDA for vitamin C, you won't contract scurvy. The board even pads the number to ensure that, even if you just barely meet its recommendation, you will still consume enough of any given nutrient. You only need 10 to 12 milligrams a day of vitamin C to ward off scurvy, but the RDA is 60 milligrams because that amount keeps blood levels of vitamin C in balance. In other words, the board factors in absorption levels and nutrient losses through cooking and other factors when it makes an RDA recommendation.

When setting the RDAs, the Food and Nutrition Board also takes a person's size and diet into account. Since, for example, infants do not need the same amount of nutrients as adult men, the board divides the RDAs along age and sex lines. In fact, 17 different groups of people can find RDAs for 26 different nutrients. Males are divided into five groups: ages 11 to 14, 15 to 18, 19 to 24, 25 to 50, and 51-plus.

Give Us This Day Our Daily Value

Sounds way too complicated, doesn't it? Well, the Food and Drug Administration agrees with you. So around 1994, it simplified matters. Rather than slicing up the population into so many sex and age categories, it came up with just a few categories based on a person's daily caloric needs. The typical food label today lists either one or two sets of Daily Values, as these new amounts are called: the daily nutrient needs for a person needing 2,000 calories a day, and the needs for a 2,500-calorie kind of guy.

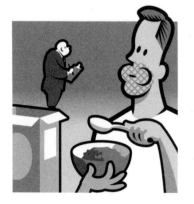

Daily Values are reported two ways. One is the actual amount of the nutrient needed, in micrograms, milligrams, or whatever. This is often the same as or very close to the RDA. But the big innovation was the other, newer reporting method. This was to give a *percentage* of your day's needs that a food provides for each nutrient. Here's an example: An average adult man should consume 2,500 calories a day to fuel his body properly. His Daily Value for vitamin C is 60 milligrams. If the man eats an orange, he gets 69.7 milligrams of vitamin C, which is 116 percent of the Daily Value. Meanwhile, a serving of marinara sauce has 16 milligrams of vitamin C, and thus meets 27 percent of his Daily Value.

Daily Values are listed as percentages on the labels of vitamin and mineral bottles and all packaged foods, instead of RDAs, because it is easier to deal with percentages than having to remember actual amounts for all those nutrients. For that reason, we'll use Daily Values for virtually all of the nutrients we discuss in this book.

The Food and Nutrition Board continues to meet every five or six years to review the studies and publish new RDAs, which then have an impact on the Daily Values, since scientists, doctors, and researchers are always finding out new things about vitamins and minerals. In fact, we are now on our 10th set of RDA guidelines.

The Daily Values are set at a level you should be able to achieve through eating a balanced diet. So if you basically follow the Food Guide Pyramid, eating more grains, fruits, and vegetables than dairy foods, meats, and sweets, you probably fulfill the Daily Values. But if you smoke cigarettes (which can deplete your stores of vitamin C), drink alcohol (which can impair the use of vitamins and minerals), or spend much of your life in the fast-food lane of your local burger joint, then there's a good chance that you don't always get the minimum levels you need.

And that's an important point to keep in mind: These numbers are intended only as guidelines for what the *average* person should consume in a day. Government agencies use the

Reading the Label

Take off your thinking cap. We're going to make it easy for you to figure out how to understand all that stuff you see on vitamin and food nutrition labels.

Milligram—$\frac{1}{1,000}$ gram (1,000 milligrams equal 1 gram). Abbreviated as mg.

Microgram—$\frac{1}{1,000,000}$ gram (1,000,000 micrograms equal 1 gram). Abbreviated as mcg.

International unit—An arbitrary standard of measurement used for vitamins A, D, and E. It has no obvious equivalents in milligrams or micrograms. Abbreviated as IU.

Recommended Dietary Allowance—The amount of a vitamin or mineral that a healthy person should get in one day. Broken down by age groups and gender. Abbreviated as RDA.

Daily Value—A simpler government standard that lets you know what percentage of recommended nutrients are in foods and supplements. It's always listed in the right-hand column of a product's nutrition label. Abbreviated as DV.

RDAs and their corresponding Daily Values as nutritional guidelines to provide adequate intakes for large groups of people, such as prisoners, schoolchildren, and the armed forces.

For example, while the Daily Value for vitamin C is 60 milligrams, early vitamin C pioneer Dr. Linus Pauling took 12,000 milligrams of C daily. That's 200 times the amount that most Americans are told to consume.

Dr. Pauling thought that vitamin C and other nutrients can be used to fight a large spectrum of health problems, not just deficiency diseases. He believed that vitamins and minerals can help prevent illnesses such as cancer and the common cold.

The question then becomes: Do you need to supplement your healthy diet with vitamin and mineral tablets? And if so, how can you do it safely?

What a Man Really Needs

The Keys to the Health and Happiness Club

Among the top killers of adult men are heart disease, cancer, stroke, and motor vehicle accidents, according to the National Center for Health Statistics. All of these, including accidents, can be affected by the foods you eat and the liquids you drink. While the relationship of fatty foods to heart disease and of alcohol to car accidents has been well-documented, good nutrition alters health in many less obvious, but equally important, ways. You need good nutrition to live long and live well.

For instance, researchers have found that if two men have oral surgery on the same day, the guy who eats a balanced, healthy diet will heal more quickly. And it comes down to something as simple as eating an orange instead of a Mounds bar.

If you've turned the corner on 40 and notice that your eyesight isn't what it used to be, don't blame age. Look at what's on your plate. When researchers looked at the possible causes of age-related macular degeneration (ARMD)—which, in layman's terms, means starting to have blurred vision as you get older—they found that those who increased their levels of the antioxidants selenium, beta-carotene, and vitamins C and E halted the progression of ARMD.

The point is that while vitamins and minerals were first thought to only fight off deficiency diseases such as anemia and rickets, we now know that they improve our quality of life as well. The ap-

propriate use of vitamins and minerals can improve many health characteristics, such as energy, mental sharpness, and some everyday aches and pains, says Dr. Cathy Kapica of Finch University of Health Sciences/Chicago Medical School.

Making Smart Choices

A healthy lifestyle is really nothing more than the composite of the dozens of small, seemingly insignificant choices you make each day. We're not about to tell you that no cheeseburger will ever again cross your lips or that you can't enjoy a cold beer on a hot summer day. If you gag at the mere whiff of brussels sprouts, we sure aren't going to tell you to hold your nose and choke 'em down anyway. The key is to arm yourself with nutritional knowledge and then make smart choices so that your body gets what it needs. If you do, when you and your best friend are standing around the shuffleboard court in 30 to 40 years, you might be the one without glasses, the one who still has sex, and the one who can follow the bingo game without asking, "What number did they just call?"

Not only that, but you may also be happier and healthier starting today. Here's how.

Trust Mother Nature. There's a good reason why they call vitamin pills supplements and not replacements. "Guys want to know if they can eat whatever they want and just take a supplement to get their vitamins and minerals. But the answer is no. You have to eat right," says Dr. Kapica.

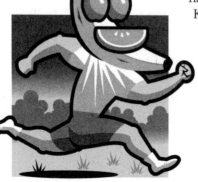

Your best source of nutrients is always food. "We know that we need certain vitamins, but there are other nutrients out there that are necessary for good health that scientists don't know about yet," Dr. Kapica says. "Relying on a supplement that has been created by researchers is only as good as the most current study, and that's not nearly as smart as relying on Mother Nature."

That's because science is still figuring out all the amazing things that vitamins and minerals do for you. For example, manganese is now considered an essential mineral because of the role it plays in numerous bodily functions. Your body uses manganese to release energy from mitochondria, part of what makes up your fast-twitch and slow-twitch muscle fibers. So even if you eat sufficient amounts of protein and fatty acids, without manganese your body would struggle to run and jump during a basketball game. No manganese, no effortless layup. While humans don't need basketball to survive, you, in particular, may consider it one element of your perfect life.

Keep your balance. You have no problem popping some Tums antacid tablets to get calcium. You even buy the orange juice with added antioxidants. But eat a tomato? No way. Broccoli? Forget about it. And you just can't seem to remember to take that mineral supplement to make sure that you get your magnesium. The problem is that missing one nutrient can have a domino effect on others.

For example, vitamin D is added to milk because its presence can increase calcium absorption by up to 30 percent. Without vitamin D, the calcium you absorb would just be chalk in your intestines. It isn't enough to simply get most of your vitamins and minerals; you have to get all of them.

And, you have to get them in the right amounts. Like calories, vitamins and minerals must be used in balance. Just as too many calories will make you fat and too few will cause fatigue, too many vitamins can cause just as much of a problem as too few.

For example, getting your Daily Value of

Terms of Confusion

Okay, you understand Daily Values, micrograms, milligrams, international units, and the other standard information relating to vitamins and minerals. Then, you pick up a supplement bottle and are confronted by a bunch of terms you've never heard before. Here's a quick glossary defining some of the most common terms you're likely to encounter.

d-alpha-tocopherol: **The natural form of vitamin E.**

dl-alpha-tocopherol: **Synthetic form of vitamin E.**

Dietary supplement: **A pill, capsule, tablet, or liquid that contains at least one of the following: a vitamin, a mineral, an herb, or similar nutritional substances. Includes such products as ginseng, garlic, fish oils, and psyllium.**

Potency: **Any vitamin or mineral in a nutritional supplement at levels well above the 100 percent Recommended Dietary Allowance.**

Provitamin: **A substance that can be converted into a vitamin by the body. Beta-carotene is a provitamin, or precursor, of vitamin A.**

Retinol equivalent (RE): **A unit of measurement for vitamin A and its various forms (1 RE equals 1 microgram of retinol or 6 micrograms of beta-carotene).**

Tocopherol equivalent (TE): **A unit of measurement for the vitamin E content of food (1 TE equals 1 milligram of d-alpha-tocopherol).**

USP: **Stands for the U.S. Pharmacopeia, an independent nonprofit and nongovernmental organization that establishes legally enforceable standards for drugs and supplements.**

magnesium may ease allergic reactions because magnesium relieves bronchospasms, or constricted airways. But don't think that loading up on magnesium will leave you wheeze-free. It's more likely to leave you with diarrhea. The moral: Just because a little of a vitamin or mineral is good doesn't mean that a lot is better.

Balance doesn't have to be as complicated as it sounds. Besides eating a well-balanced diet, you can get added insurance by taking the right multivitamin/mineral supplement, says Joanne Curran-Celentano, R.D., Ph.D., associate professor of nutrition and food sciences at the University of New Hampshire in Durham. But supplements should be just a form of insurance for days when you don't eat well or if you're under a lot of stress, she says. Although they're easy, cost very little money, and have little risk, the best form of insurance, says Dr. Curran-Celentano, is just eating right most days and reducing overall stress.

A man's multivitamin/mineral supplement should have 100 percent of the Daily Value for most of the nutrients, plus extra E and C. Most men should not take a supplement with iron, says Dr. Curran-Celentano.

Know what you need—and what you don't. Besides iron, there are a handful of other vitamins and minerals that men don't need to supplement. If you find more than 100 percent of the Daily Value of vitamins A, D, or K; biotin; phosphorus; copper; or iron in your supplement, throw them out and buy a new one. These are easily absorbed and stored vitamins and minerals. Your body doesn't need excess amounts, and in some cases, too much can be a dangerous thing.

Living Right

Just as vitamin and mineral supplements are no substitute for a healthy diet, they can't make up for unhealthy lifestyle habits. "Since the turn of the century, we've seen a decline in the incidences of heart disease in this country. But that may not have anything to do with an increased use of supplements," says Christopher

The Future

Some nutrition researchers think that the current Daily Values should be bumped up because the numbers only tell us how much we need to maintain nutritional health, not how much we need for maximum benefits. The Food and Nutrition Board has been considering whether to present the idea of chronic disease into the equations of the RDAs.

In fact, a special subcommittee of the Food and Nutrition Board began meeting in 1993 to review the studies on vitamin and mineral intake. "The committee may come out with new values that would help a health-conscious consumer make better food choices," says Mona Calvo, Ph.D., a member of the clinical research and review staff for the Food and Drug Administration in Washington, D.C.

The board is moving to create three categories: The Estimated Average Requirement, the Daily Recommended Intakes, and a number that reflects the Upper Level of Safety, or the amount that could possibly prove toxic, Dr. Calvo says. These terms, regardless of whether they are finally adopted by the board, should prove valuable.

- The Estimated Average Requirement would reflect the average amount a person needs to consume in order to avoid any deficiency disease. In the case

Gardner, Ph.D., a nutrition researcher at Stanford University's Center for Research in Disease Prevention. "It reflects changes in our lifestyles and the environment."

In other words, the top killers of men these days cannot be stopped by popping a magic dose of vitamins and minerals. While vitamin C may help the body mitigate the effects of cigarette smoking, it can't undo much of the damage that smoke in your lungs can generate. Likewise, people have been taking beta-carotene supplements to help prevent heart dis-

of vitamin C, for example, that would most likely be lower than its current Daily Value of 60 milligrams.

- **The Daily Recommended Intake would reflect the amounts that have been shown to fight other illnesses. For example, research has found that vitamin C may help prevent shortness of breath caused by asthma and bronchitis. Likewise, another study found that taking 2,000 milligrams (or 33 times the Daily Value) helps open blocked arteries. The Daily Recommended Intake would reflect the highest level at which a vitamin or mineral has been safely shown to provide disease protection.**

- **The Upper Level of Safety would caution consumers against the amount of each vitamin and mineral that is considered dangerous to consume. For example, taking more than 1,200 milligrams of vitamin C at any given time may lead to diarrhea and possibly kidney stone problems.**

The committee looking at the changes has divided the nutrients into nine subcategories. The first group to be reviewed and revised includes calcium, vitamin D, phosphorus, magnesium, and fluoride—all bone-building materials. These vitamins and minerals are being studied together so that the board can organize a nutritional fight against osteoporosis, a disease that afflicts both men and women.

would choose the vitamin."

For one thing, says Dr. Gardner, there are a lot of side effects to drugs that vitamins don't have. And second, there is often less risk associated with taking supplements. "In most cases, you're wasting your money by taking a supplement if you aren't lacking in it because extra doesn't do you any good," he says. In a few cases, overdoing it with supplements can even have severe consequences. For instance, regularly taking large quantities of vitamin A (more than 50,000 international units a day) could cause blurred vision, hair loss, enlarged liver and spleen or even death.

So do your homework. If heart disease runs in your family, ask your physician if a vitamin E supplement will help. If you're in recovery from alcohol or drug addiction, ask about including antioxidants and a multimineral supplement. If you are a diabetic, talk to your doctor about chromium.

"Unfortunately, some doctors and pharmacists aren't well-trained in nutrition," says Dr. Curran-Celentano. In general, dietitians will tell you to eat better before they will recommend supplementation. "Ask questions and do research into your illness to see which diets best helped other sufferers and if there is a record of supplementation use associated with it. Then ask your physician if any changes that you'd like to make will interfere with the actions you're already taking or with your medication."

On the flip side, if you're on medication, find out if it interferes with your body's use of certain vitamins and minerals. Both over-the-counter and prescription drugs, including antacids, antibiotics, and tranquilizers, can diminish your body's ability to utilize certain nutrients. If that's the case, a supplement might be in order while you're on the medicine.

ease, and research is now showing that at best they haven't helped at all, Dr. Gardner says.

There still are a lot of experts who don't believe in the use of vitamin and mineral supplements, including Dr. Gardner, who advocates a balanced diet and lots of exercise. "I'm totally opposed to using supplements in place of a nutritious diet," he says. Although Dr. Gardner cautions that no vitamin can replace a prescribed drug, he admits, "If I had a choice between taking a medicine to fight heart disease and a vitamin that did the same thing, I

The Ultimate Program

For Guys Who Live to the Max

While the Daily Values are designed to keep everyone healthy at the most basic level, people now want their vitamins and minerals to go beyond the minimum requirement. We want our nutrients to help us be active, work hard, combat stress, and prevent illnesses such as cancer and heart disease.

So we asked two of the leading experts in the field—Dr. Shari Lieberman, co-author of *The Real Vitamin and Mineral Book*, and Alexander Schauss, Ph.D., author of *Minerals, Trace Elements, and Human Health*—to come up with recommendations that will help men live life to the fullest.

"Scientific literature has consistently demonstrated a protective effect for people using supplements," Dr. Lieberman says. "Reports of toxicity problems have been very rare."

The table below, which lists optimal vitamin and mineral intakes, is divided into three sections: one for nutrients that you can easily get from food; one for nutrients that you probably need to supplement; and one for nutrients that you may want to consider supplementing. The goal is to devise a sensible vitamin and mineral program for men that offers optimal, but safe, levels that bestow maximum disease

Vitamin/ Mineral	Daily Value for Men	Suggested Optimal Amount	Toxicity and Symptoms	
No Supplementation Necessary				
Vitamin A	5,000 IU	10,000 IU	50,000 IU: Dry skin, nausea, headaches, fatigue, irritability, liver damage	
Beta-carotene	No Daily Value	25,000 IU	None known	
Vitamin D	400 IU	400 IU	1,000 IU: Loss of appetite, headache, excessive thirst	
Vitamin K	80 mcg	80 mcg	In rare instances—primarily with infants and pregnant women—can result when water-soluble substitutes are prescribed. Can result in jaundice or brain damage.	
Biotin	300 mcg	300 mcg	None known	
Boron	No Daily Value	3 mg	Under investigation, but currently thought to be 3 mg. Symptoms unknown.	

protection and health benefits.

In the table, the category "Toxicity and Symptoms" lists the levels at which harmful side effects occur. However, some people will experience problems at significantly lower levels. That's why you'll notice cautions in chapters throughout this book advising that you consult a physician before exceeding certain levels, even though they fall below the amounts in the "Toxicity and Symptoms" category. Also, pay careful attention to the abbreviated amounts for each vitamin and mineral. Mg is short for milligrams, which are $1/1,000$ gram. Mcg stands for micrograms, or $1/1,000,000$ gram. That's a big difference, so take the time to be sure.

The Food and Nutrition Board (which sets the Daily Values and Recommended Dietary Allowances) doesn't use the word optimal, perhaps because it's not an easily definable term and is somewhat relative. However, the National Institutes of Health used the term in a 1994 paper on calcium and osteoporosis. That was one of the first times an official paper has used it.

Does this mean that everyone should start popping vitamins at the highest dosage they can find? Absolutely not. The difference between the government recommendations and the optimal levels varies tremendously depending on the vitamin or mineral involved. Some, like vitamin K, remain the same. But others, like vitamins C and E, increase dramatically. So it's important to understand that megadosing and optimal levels are not one and the same. "Megadosing technically means 10 or more times the Recommended Dietary Allowance," says Dr. Joanne Curran-Celentano of the University of New Hampshire.

Uses	Food Sources
Helps maintain good vision and healthy skin. Supports the immune system and promotes growth.	Fish and animal foods
Helps protect against cancer, cardiovascular disease, and cataracts.	Carrots, sweet potatoes, spinach, fresh parsley
Helps absorption of calcium and phosphorus for strong bones.	Fortified milk, eggs, fish and fish oils
Plays major role in blood clotting.	Green, leafy vegetables; milk; eggs
Helps metabolize fat, protein, and carbohydrates.	Peanut butter, wheat germ, liver, eggs
Helps metabolize calcium and magnesium. Enhances mental alertness.	Apples, pears

(continued)

Vitamin/ Mineral	Daily Value for Men	Suggested Optimal Amount	Toxicity and Symptoms	
No Supplementation Necessary—Continued				
Copper	2 mg	2 mg	10 mg: Vomiting, diarrhea	
Fluoride	No Daily Value	4 mg	20 mg per day over many years: Teeth discoloration, nausea, chest pain, vomiting	
Iodine	150 mcg	150 mcg	2,000 mcg: Enlargement of thyroid gland	
Iron	10 mg	15 mg	75 mg: Loss of body hair, lethargy, impotence	
Manganese	2 mg	10 mg	Usually occurs from inhalation of pollutants, not dietary intake	
Molybdenum	75 mcg	75 mcg	250 mcg: Diarrhea, anemia	
Phosphorus	1,000 mg	1,000 mg	A calcium-to-phosphorus ratio lower than 1 to 2: Lowering of blood calcium levels to detriment of teeth and bones	
Sodium	2,400 mg	2,400 mg	None because kidneys excrete excess	
Supplementation Strongly Recommended				
Vitamin B$_6$	2 mg	15 mg	100 mg per day over extended time period: Depression, fatigue, numbness of feet, hands, mouth	
Vitamin C	60 mg	1,000 mg	2,000 mg: Headache, insomnia, hot flashes, rashes, diarrhea	
Vitamin E	30 IU	400 IU	900 IU: Digestive tract discomfort	

Uses	Food Sources
Works with iron to make hemoglobin.	Legumes, grains, seeds, liver
Helps form bones and teeth. Helps prevent tooth decay.	Fluoridated drinking water, tea, seafood
Helps regulate growth, development, and metabolic rate.	Iodized salt, seafood, bread, dairy products
Transports and stores oxygen in red blood cells. Helps with hormone production. Assists the immune system. Enhances thinking abilities.	Beef, cream of wheat cereal, baked potatoes, pumpkin seeds, clams
Development of the skeleton and connective tissue. Crucial to normal brain function.	Nuts, tea, whole grains, cereals
Moderates excretion of uric acid and sulfate.	Milk and milk products, beans, meats, cereals
Numerous bone, muscle, and energy functions.	Nonfat yogurt, salmon, skim milk, chicken, oatmeal, tomatoes
Essential to nerve transmission and muscle contraction.	Salt, soy sauce, processed foods
Helps maintain healthy hair, skin, eyes, nerves, and digestion.	Whole grains; green, leafy vegetables; beans; nuts; poultry; fish
Helps form collagen, which strengthens blood vessel walls and forms scar tissue. Also strengthens resistance against infection.	Oranges, cranberry juice, cantaloupe, broccoli, peppers, pink grapefruit, kiwifruit
Fights heart disease and some cancers.	Vegetable and nut oils, sunflower seeds, whole grains, wheat germ, spinach

(continued)

Vitamin/ Mineral	Daily Value for Men	Suggested Optimal Amount	Toxicity and Symptoms	
Supplementation Strongly Recommended—Continued				
Calcium	1,000 mg	Up to age 65: 1,000 mg Age 65+: 1,500 mg	None known	
Chromium	120 mcg	200 mcg	Unknown as a nutrition disorder	
Folic acid	400 mcg	400 mcg	Levels of more than 400 mcg can mask B_{12} deficiencies.	
Magnesium	400 mg	500 mg	None known in people with normal renal function	
Niacin	20 mg	30 mg	200 mg: Diarrhea, heartburn, dizziness, fainting, itching, sweating	
Potassium	3,500 mg	3,500 mg	18,000 mg: Results from overuse of potassium salts, not overeating foods high in potassium. Can result in muscle weakness, vomiting, heart failure.	
Riboflavin	1.7 mg	2.5 mg	None known	
Selenium	70 mcg	200 mcg	1,000 mcg per day over extended period of time: Loss of hair and nails, skin lesions, tooth decay, nervous system disorders	
Thiamin	1.5 mg	10 mg	None known	
Zinc	15 mg	15 mg	100 mg: Raised cholesterol, diarrhea, fever, fatigue, dizziness, reproductive failure	
Supplementation Should Be Considered				
Vitamin B_{12}	6 mcg	6 mcg	None known	

Uses	Food Sources
Builds strong teeth and bones. Healthy growth.	Milk, yogurt, cheese
May help prevent adult-onset diabetes. Metabolizes glucose.	Brewer's yeast, sugar, meats, whole grains, syrups
Helps make DNA. Assists in cell reproduction. Reduces elevated homocysteine.	Asparagus, cereals, pinto beans, navy beans, spinach
Works in metabolism and nerve functions.	Meats; poultry; dairy products; cereal; dark green, leafy vegetables
Used in energy metabolism. Supports health of skin, nervous system, and digestive system.	Poultry, tuna, most meats, many cereals
Balances electrolyte levels. Keeps nerves firing and muscles contracting.	Bananas, potatoes, beans, spinach
Supports vision and skin health. Helps with energy conversion.	Fortified and enriched foods, milk products, spinach, meats
May fight cancer and heart disease.	Seafood, meats, grains, Brazil nuts
Supports appetite and nerve function.	Fortified and enriched foods, pork, wheat germ
Strengthens immune system. Involved in taste perception, wound healing, and sperm production. Essential for brain function.	Red meats, poultry, eggs, oysters
Involved in DNA production. Protects nerve fibers.	Beef, fish, milk

Getting What You Need from Food

Tapping Into Nature's Nutrient Storehouse

Want to give less money to your doctor next year? Then give more money to your grocer. Economic research has revealed that if Americans ate more foods high in vitamins C and E and beta-carotene, our national health care costs would decrease by 25 percent—for cardiovascular disease alone. Cancer costs would drop by 16 to 30 percent, and cataract costs would plummet by 50 percent. It's an alchemist's dream: turning carrots into dollars.

"You can fulfill the Recommended Dietary Allowances for vitamins and minerals by following the Food Guide Pyramid," says Keith-Thomas Ayoob, R.D., Ed.D., spokesman for the American Dietetic Association in Chicago, director of nutrition services at the Rose F. Kennedy Children's Evaluation and Rehabilitation Center, and assistant professor of pediatric medicine at Albert Einstein College of Medicine, both in New York City. "There are times when vitamin supplementation can be necessary and appropriate, but if you eat a proper diet, not only will you meet your nutrient needs but you'll probably exceed them."

That's because vitamins and minerals are only the tip of the iceberg, nutritionally speaking. No amount of supplementation can replace a good diet, nor can it fix the damage an unhealthy diet can do, in both

the short and long term. In fact, trying to replace food with supplements can actually do more harm than good. Throughout the rest of this chapter, we'll discuss the variety of foods you need to eat every day—fruits and vegetables, whole grains, dairy products, meats, and fats, sweets, and oils. If that list sounds familiar, it should: It's on the official Food Guide Pyramid.

Fruits and Vegetables

Scientists have discovered that plant foods—fruits and vegetables—seem to be as important for what we don't know about them as for what we do. "A natural food is much more than the sum of its known nutrients," says Barbara Klein, Ph.D., professor of food science and human nutrition at the University of Illinois in Urbana-Champaign. "We know a lot about vitamins and minerals, but we don't know a lot about the other compounds that are present in plants. Our knowledge is not sufficient to warrant taking supplements and not eating well."

In fact, researchers have found that vegetables and fruit contain chemicals, dubbed phytochemicals, that help protect against cancer and other diseases. Among the handful of phytochemicals that have been isolated so far are capsaicin (found in peppers), flavonoids (berries, citrus fruits, and yams), allylic sulfide (onions and garlic), and indole-3-carbinol (cauliflower and cabbage).

Like vitamins and minerals, phytochemicals lose some of their protective powers when they're isolated from the foods they come in.

For example, just a few years ago, researchers found that men with cancer had less beta-carotene in their blood than those without cancer. At first it seemed that beta-carotene alone could block the development of cancer, but when researchers looked further into the issue, they found something else entirely.

"It turned out that taking

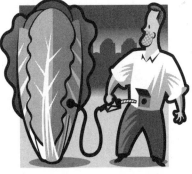

beta-carotene supplements actually had an adverse effect, because when you isolate beta-carotene down to a pill, something important that appears in the food is removed. But we're still not completely sure about what it is," says Dr. Christopher Gardner of Stanford University's Center for Research in Disease Prevention. Researchers are still learning how various chemicals work together to offer protection against disease. And their discoveries spark a sense of awe.

Nature packages foods in a miraculous way. For instance, while a mineral pill might contain more iron than a tomato, the tomato has vitamin C, which aids the body's absorption of that iron.

Likewise, the tomato will have other nutrients that can help your health. For instance, a study found that a carotenoid called lycopene has a more protective effect against prostate cancer than both vitamin A and beta-carotene. Lycopene is most commonly found in tomatoes and tomato-based foods, such as tomato sauce—a food, not a vitamin or mineral supplement. So, you'd have to take at least three supplements—vitamin C, iron, and lycopene—to equal just the known protective nutrients found in tomatoes and tomato products.

Even nutritionists who endorse supplementation agree that people taking vitamin and mineral tablets should do so in addition to a low-fat diet that features the recommended servings of fruits and vegetables. "A vitamin pill can't compensate for a diet that's loaded with fat or low in fruits and vegetables because there are thousands of plant compounds that may help reduce the risk of cancer and heart disease," says Bonnie Liebman, licensed nutritionist and director of nutrition for the Center for Science in the Public Interest in Washington, D.C.

Federal surveys have consistently shown, however, that 60 percent of what Americans eat comes from animal-based foods, with the remaining 40 percent coming from plant sources. The ratio should be precisely the opposite, experts say.

Whole Grains

Talk to any nutritionist and they'll sing the praises of plants, but not just fruits and vegetables. The next group of foods to add to your shopping cart is whole grains.

"Whole wheat, oats, barley, rye, millet, brown rice, and corn are all whole grains," Dr. Klein says. "During processing, they have as little removed as possible to make them palatable." In other words, while the wheat no longer has those fuzzy things on the top, all that's taken off during processing is the hull. What's left (after processing) is the grain with the bran or the germ attached.

So, while oatmeal is a whole grain, traditional spaghetti isn't. (In fact, spaghetti, as we know it, contains all of the starch but little of the vitamins and minerals in the grain.) Rye bread contains whole grains, but white bread doesn't. Wheatena is a whole grain, but farina isn't. The more refined the flour, the less nutritious the food, Dr. Klein says.

Dairy Products

Guys don't drink enough milk, and that's bad because it's an extremely nutrient-dense food. (Sorry, but it's not true that you get extra fiber by drinking it straight from the carton.) In fact, all the vitamins as well as six minerals have been detected in cow milk. Of course, the most obvious nutrient identified with milk is calcium.

Two glasses (8 ounces each) of milk will provide about 60 percent of the Daily Value for calcium. About 95 percent of the milk supply in the United States is fortified with vitamin D, which helps the body absorb the calcium found in the milk. However, even though it's great to get calcium through milk, it's only worth it, calorically speaking, if you're drinking low-fat or skim milk. Whole milk is just too high in fat.

The ways in which milk is made into other dairy products also affects the food's level of calcium. For instance, one serving of Cheddar cheese has more than twice the calcium as a serving of cottage cheese. The drawback is that it also has four times the calories. However, it is still more nutrient-smart to consume a small amount of Cheddar.

Meat

Unless you're following a vegetarian diet, low-fat meats can still have an honored place on your plate—though probably not quite as large—because many of the vitamins and minerals in meat are more bioavailable than those in plant food. That means that your body absorbs them better. (For more on absorption, see Enrichment and Fortification on page 24.)

"It's not an issue of never eating meat," Liebman says. "It's about how often you eat it. Your diet should be largely plant-based." A plant-based diet can cut your risk of cancer, heart disease, stroke, and diabetes, she adds.

Surveys show that only half of all Americans eat fruit every day and more than 20 percent consume no milk products. But 25 percent of all Americans eat fried potatoes on any given day. "The problem is that a meat-and-potatoes diet usually means that a man isn't eating fruits and vegetables," Liebman says. "If a guy wants his steak, he should think of the salad as the main course and the meat as a side dish."

Or, think of meat as what you eat when you go out to dinner on the weekends rather than your everyday evening meal. If you have meat for lunch and dinner, cut back to once a day, Liebman advises.

Fats

Hopefully, there's hardly any room left in your stomach. But if there is, you get to have a treat. And most people choose fat-laden treats.

Sneaking Produce In

Surely, we all look forward with great anticipation to the annual observance of "Sneak Some Zucchini onto Your Neighbors' Porch Night" each August. But we'd be a lot better off if we concentrated more on sneaking some zucchini and other fruits and vegetables onto our own plates every day.

On average, American men eat three servings of fruits and vegetables a day. But they should be getting a minimum of five servings and really ought to shoot for nine.

We're not about to suggest that you change your diet completely. But by making a few simple substitutions, you can easily boost your consumption of fruit and vegetables without feeling like you've just been put out to pasture.

"One of the best ideas is to add a can of vegetable soup to your diet or some frozen vegetables to your pasta dishes, and do it every day," says Dr. Barbara Klein of the University of Illinois. "Make it a soup that's noncreamy, or uses low-fat dairy, and is low in sodium." Here are some suggestions: tomato, corn chowder, cream of spinach or broccoli made with skim milk, or any soup or stew with lots of vegetables. Hot soup is also a great food for weight loss, since it fills you up on fewer calories.

Another good place to start is to add a side salad to your lunch, especially if you're eating it instead of an order of french fries. Here are some other ideas to sneak a bit more produce into your diet.

The Food Guide Pyramid recommends that you eat fat "sparingly," says Dr. Klein, which means that if you eat any animal products, such as meats, you don't need to add much fat to anything during the day. "That source alone probably fills your recommended intake," she says.

So put down the butter knife. If you

Breakfast

- Raisins or another dried fruit in your oatmeal
- Fresh fruit spread with no added sugar on your toast
- A banana
- Sautéed apple slices to go with low-cholesterol eggs

Lunch

- Rice with mixed vegetables and shrimp at a Chinese restaurant (ask for a white sauce rather than a higher-sodium brown sauce, and no monosodium glutamate, or MSG)
- Mushrooms, tomatoes, green peppers, and spinach on your pizza
- Canned fruit for dessert

Dinner

- A baked potato with salsa instead of butter or sour cream
- A bag of frozen mixed vegetables (without a sauce) mixed with pasta while it cooks and dressed with basil and olive oil
- Onions, peppers, and zucchini in your spaghetti sauce or hidden in your lasagna
- Lots of onions and red peppers in your chili

Snacks

- Yogurt with fruit but no sugar added
- Applesauce (unsweetened) or other canned fruit
- Salsa with baked, not fried, chips
- Dried apricots
- Frozen grapes (on the stem)

salad dressing. "If you have a choice, don't use fat," Dr. Klein says.

Smart Eating

If you focus on getting all your vitamins and minerals, not to mention your carotenoids and phytochemicals, you'll have a full plate as well as a full belly. There might not be a lot of room left for nonnutritious items.

When it comes to food, Dr. Klein says, variety is indeed the spice of life. "There's no single food or group of foods that by itself is perfect," she says. "We have many nutritional needs that we know of and some that we don't know. Eating a balanced diet means that you should eat a wide variety of foods." So while there's tons of proof that fruits and vegetables can help prevent cancer, they're not the only foods that provide vitamins and minerals.

"Remember that you can eat a pizza or hamburger for breakfast and still have a balanced diet," says Dr. Klein. "You just want to make sure that there's a large distribution among the kinds of food you eat."

In fact, you could take a tip from the Japanese. Their government recommends that its citizens eat 30 "foodstuffs" each day, which roughly corresponds to the highest number of recommended servings in the Food Guide Pyramid.

And don't think that all this eating means that you'll never take supplements. In fact, just the opposite is true. Studies have shown that people who take supplements eat more servings of fruits and vegetables than those who don't eat well. And you know what other group you'll join? Those with higher personal incomes and more education. They, too, eat better and take more supplements.

must, lean toward oils rather than margarine or butter. "We have a lot of hidden fat in our diets, particularly with fast food," Dr. Klein says. "It's not the hamburger that's killing us. It's the special sauce, to say nothing of the french fries."

Aim for 2 tablespoons or less a day of oils (preferably those high in monounsaturates, such as olive oil), which translates into a serving of

Enrichment and Fortification

Understanding the Jellybean Rule

There's vitamin D in your milk, niacin in your bread, and iodine in your salt. And have you looked at orange juice lately? You can now choose among juices with extra calcium, a cocktail of vitamins A, C, and E, or just plain-old no pulp.

These are all examples of enrichment and fortification, two of the reasons why the United States has such a healthy and nutritious food supply. While the words are used interchangeably, they both refer to the addition of specific nutrients to food.

Enrichment and fortification are inexpensive and efficient ways to ensure that people get at least the minimum amount of necessary vitamins and minerals. Some nutrients are added to food because they are lost in processing (such as the B vitamins in white bread), while others are added because they aid the absorption of other nutrients already found in a food (such as adding vitamin D to milk, which helps the absorption of calcium).

"Fortification of foods generates controversy among food technologists," says James Giese, associate editor of *Food Technology* magazine. One problem is that manufacturers could add vitamins and minerals to nutritionally insignificant foods—such as jellybeans—so that people who live on junk food would think that they are getting at least some nutrients. But U.S. Food and Drug Administration guidelines discourage

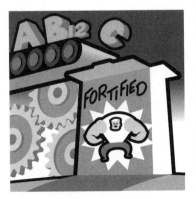

adding nutrients to foods of little nutritional value. This conundrum is known informally as the jellybean rule, says Giese.

The Prize in the Cereal Box

The easiest place to see the impact of fortification is to look at the nutritional information on the side of a cereal box.

"Breakfast provides about 25 percent of daily calories for most Americans," says Dr. Joanne Curran-Celentano of the University of New Hampshire. Therefore, most cereals are fortified at those levels. "Eating a fortified cereal is one way to help reach your Daily Values for some nutrients," Dr. Curran-Celentano says.

The vitamins used in cereal are the same vitamins you get in a supplement. For example, look on the side of a box of Kellogg's All-Bran and you'll see, listed among the ingredients, pyridoxine hydrochloride or vitamin B_6, just as you will on a bottle of Centrum.

"Fortified breakfast cereals provide a more nutrient-dense breakfast than many other breakfast foods, including home fries and eggs," Dr. Curran-Celentano says. "Eating a high-fiber cereal will make the meal even more healthful."

There is a catch, though: The presence of fiber inhibits the absorption of some vitamins and minerals. Added to this problem are the additions of sugar and salt to almost all fortified cereals. All-Bran's second ingredient is sugar, followed by corn syrup and malt flavoring—all sweetening agents. Some cereals are high in sodium, too (it's All-Bran's fifth ingredient).

In some ways, cereals look more like a dessert than an entrée, but Dr. Curran-Celentano says that could be a good thing. "A lot of people are inclined to overeat after dinner," she says. "And what they eat are traditionally snack foods, which are low in nutrients but high in calories. Cereals, especially high-fiber ones, can be a good replacement for an evening snack. If you're careful about which cereal you choose and eat the proper serving size, eating cereal as a snack rather than potato chips or ice cream will cut down your calorie intake but still give you a rich amount of vitamins and minerals."

While a fortified cereal boasts a long list of vitamins and minerals, it is only part of a healthy diet. It's true that you'll get a well-rounded amount of nutrients in a fortified cereal, but you won't get the phytochemicals found in whole foods. Even cereal companies suggest that you complement their foods with at least a glass of orange juice or some fruit. Foods like these that come by their nutrients naturally contain components other than vitamins and minerals that are important for your body's nutritional needs.

The New Wave

"The government used to order fortification solely to fight deficiency diseases," says Liz Applegate, Ph.D., nutrition columnist for *Runner's World* magazine and author of *Power Foods.* "But the Food and Drug Administration has just ordered many manufacturers to fortify their foods with folic acid, and that isn't to prevent a deficiency disease, but to optimize the health of newborns, whose mothers need more folic acid." Men should benefit, too, says Dr. Applegate because folic acid seems to play a role in fighting heart disease. Folic acid will be added to all enriched grain products starting in January 1998.

Enriched and fortified foods are a good dietary supplement for people who know that they don't get enough of certain vitamins and

The Wonders of Wonder Bread

The number one selling bread in the United States is Wonder bread, a fortified product famous for "helping to build strong bodies 12 ways." Wonder bread, owned by the Interstate Bakeries Corporation, has been fortified since 1941, when it joined the government-supported bread-enrichment program. But Wonder bread is no more enriched than any enriched white flour or white bread.

Talk to some nutritionists and they may let you in on the secret of enriched white bread. Yes, it has added vitamins and minerals, but not nearly enough to equal the nutritional strength of a whole-wheat product. Processing removes several key nutrients from whole-white flour including zinc, folate (the natural form of folic acid), magnesium, and vitamin E. But the enrichment of white bread adds only five nutrients back in: thiamin, niacin, riboflavin, iron, and—starting in January 1998—folic acid.

"Half of all bread sold in the country is white bread," according to Mark Dirkes, senior vice president of marketing for Interstate Bakeries Corporation, in Kansas City, Missouri. "And we think the question of which is more nutritious is almost irrelevant. We offer a wheat bread wherever we sell Wonder, but only 25 percent of breads sold are wheat. People, especially kids, prefer white."

minerals, says Dr. Applegate. Athletes and vegetarians often don't get enough calcium and B_{12} in their diets. They would benefit from eating one meal or snack with a fortified food, such as cereal. Another good group of candidates is people who don't eat milk products either because they are lactose-intolerant or because they just don't like milk. If you don't drink milk on a regular basis, says Dr. Applegate, then calcium-fortified orange juice is a good option.

Making the Most of What You Get

Enter the Theater of the Absorb

File this under the category "Life Isn't Fair." You can swallow all the vitamins and minerals—either from food or supplements or both—that the government says you need and still miss out on the health benefits. Because the real question is not how much you consume but how much of the nutrients are absorbed by your body.

Absorption is a multistep process. Your mouth chews the food (or swallows the supplement) and the small pieces travel down, eventually settling in your small intestine. Covering the 20 feet or so of your small intestine are small cells that absorb nutrients. These cells, called microvilli, regulate the passage of each nutrient into the bloodstream.

The microvilli have enzymes in them that digest the nutrients and allow them to be absorbed by other cells within the intestines. In a sense, the microvilli are your bloodstream's traffic cops, deciding whether to wave the nutrients on to travel through the blood or to detour them along the digestive tract for excretion.

"The Recommended Dietary Allowances (RDAs) don't take absorption issues into account," says J. Cecil Smith, Ph.D., a research chemist at the U.S. Department of Agriculture's (USDA's) phytonutrients laboratory in Beltsville, Maryland. In other words, the present RDAs don't tell us how readily a nutrient can be absorbed from different foods. For example, iron is more readily absorbed—more bioavailable—from steak than from spinach. There is a push to incorporate this knowledge in future editions of the RDAs, Dr. Smith adds. That already has been done in some other countries, including the United Kingdom.

They'll Melt with You

If you're a vitamin, it all comes down to one question: What does it take to break you down? Four vitamins—A, D, E, and K—can be absorbed only with help from dietary fat, so they're known as fat-soluble. They are stored in fatty tissues and in the liver, hanging around the body until they're needed. That means that you're less likely to run short of them, but it also means that you run the risk of stockpiling too many, which can be dangerous—especially with vitamins A and D. Adults who get too much vitamin A have been known to suffer from a number of symptoms, ranging from headaches to hair loss. Getting too much vitamin D can cause appetite loss, weight loss, and nausea.

The B-complex and C vitamins dissolve in water, earning them the moniker—you guessed it—water-soluble. Only small amounts of these vitamins get stored in the body, so the odds of toxic side effects are much slimmer. However, the chances of not getting enough are that much greater.

It's the B vitamins that change the color of urine. If you have adequate stores of the vitamin in your body, then you'll pee out what you don't need. Depending on how hydrated you are, this could take anywhere from a half-hour to 4 to 6 hours.

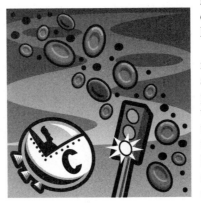

But all of this really means one thing to you: Water-soluble vitamins have to be replenished daily. Fat-soluble vitamins don't. Just be aware that large doses of fat-soluble vitamins can cause trouble because they won't be excreted as easily as their water-soluble cousins.

The Gatekeeper in Your Gut

In some cases, your body will hold on to a particular nutrient if it needs it and let it go if it doesn't. In fact, the rate of absorption of some nutrients can vary from one meal to the next. So if you've eaten iron-rich Cream of Wheat cereal for breakfast, your body may decide to forgo some of the iron found in the tofu on your salad at lunchtime.

"Each individual apparently has genetic components for absorption that he doesn't have much control over," Dr. Smith says. "But there is flexibility and a desire for homeostasis within that level. It's almost as if there's a gatekeeper within your gut who allows an appropriate level of nutrients to pass through depending on the nutritional needs of the person."

For instance, if you're deficient in iron, or anemic, your absorption level may be as high as 80 percent; but it can also be as low as 5 percent if your iron stores are high.

Bioavailability: What the Body Keeps

"Researchers are much more interested in the bioavailability of vitamins and minerals, which is not synonymous with the total amount found in the food by chemical analysis," says Dr. Smith. Bioavailability measures how much of any given nutrient the body is able to absorb from a single food or supplement. For instance, growing children absorb 75 percent of the dietary calcium in foods such as milk. But as people age, they begin to absorb less, in amounts as low as 10 percent.

Likewise, the calcium in milk is more bioavailable than the calcium in broccoli. Several factors play into that, including the presence of protein, the type of calcium found in each food, and the amount of vitamin D added to milk.

"We know that there are often large differences in the bioavailability of minerals from plant-derived foods compared to foods from animal products," Dr. Smith says. "For instance,

zinc from wheat germ is less bioavailable than flesh or seafood sources." A number of processes can affect bioavailability.

• Phytates and oxalates. These two plant fibers bind to calcium and iron, among other minerals, and carry them out of the body. Oxalates are one reason why only about 5 percent of the iron in spinach is bioavailable.

"Phytic acid is in a plant because it's a source of phosphorous required for the germinating seed," Dr. Smith says. "But phytic acid also binds zinc and inhibits its absorption." Another word for this binding process is *chelation*, pronounced "kee-LAY-shun."

• Prescription and over-the-counter drugs. For a variety of reasons, antacids, antibiotics, laxatives, and other medications can affect the body's ability to absorb certain minerals. Talk to a doctor or pharmacist about possible absorption side effects from both over-the-counter and prescription medications. Also ask if you should use a vitamin or mineral supplement while using a medication.

• Food additives. Some of the products added to foods, both natural and synthetic, affect the body's ability to use minerals. For instance, gums used to thicken processed foods bind with iron and copper, creating a nonabsorbable complex. Processed and refined foods usually have fewer nutrients than nonprocessed foods. For example, table sugar has a markedly lower mineral content than the molasses from which it is refined.

• Fiber. We're all for a high-fiber diet, but...well, think about it. You're getting that extra fiber to get stuff out of your body. Bran is rich in phytates, for example, which bind to minerals. On the other hand, bran has much higher levels of minerals overall than bleached or white flour, so it's still a better food choice than processed grains, says Dr. Cathy Kapica of Finch University of Health Sciences/Chicago Medical School.

• Metabolism problems. Diabetes, high blood pressure, anemia, and other illnesses can alter the body's balance of vitamins and minerals. Diabetes, for example, can lead to depletion of bone calcium and muscle potassium. Once again, talk to a nutritionist or physician about any illness, including temporary problems such as the flu or a cold. They may be able to advise you on dietary additions that will decrease the likelihood of deficiency problems.

• Age. As we get older, the hydrochloric acid levels in our stomachs begin to decrease, and this can impair absorption levels. At the same time, older people need to eat fewer calories because their metabolisms have slowed, yet they need the same amount of nutrients. It's hard for them to get those nutrients if they're eating less. The RDA levels do not reflect these changes, but some nutritionists believe that supplementation is important for people over the age of 50.

Increasing Absorption

There is a direct correlation between the richness of soil and the nutrient density of the food it yields. Selenium, iodine, and other minerals, for example, are found in varying levels throughout the world. Some regions in the United States have rich levels of selenium, while others have almost none.

In addition, overgrazing and intense farming as well as the use of pesticides and other chemicals in agriculture can alter the levels of nutrients in our foods. Some studies suggest that organic farming, which strives to maintain the health of the soil by building up its organic matter, rotating crops, and minimizing the use of pesticides, may produce higher yields as well as plants with higher mineral levels. One study done by a Swiss researcher found that organically grown spinach had twice as much B_{12} as conventionally grown spinach.

Get Dense

Overcooking broccoli in a big pot of boiling water renders its nutrient powers as limp as the soggy stalks you pull out of the pot. Most of the water-soluble vitamins are left in the pot of water.

Statistics show that most of us don't get anywhere near the number of vegetables that we should each day. So it certainly makes no sense to boil the vital vitamins and minerals out of the precious few we do get. Here's how to keep your vegetables dense—nutrient-dense, that is.

Watch the time. "The best way to cook vegetables is with a minimum amount of water for the shortest period of time possible," says Dr. Barbara Klein of the University of Illinois. **"Microwaving and steaming are ideal. But if you prefer the color and texture of vegetables that are boiled in water, the critical thing is to boil them for the shortest time possible."**

The shortest time possible, in this case, translates to 3 to 7 minutes because that's long enough to extract the water-soluble vitamins (all the Bs and C) from the food. The key is to aim for a texture known as tender-crisp, says Dr. Klein. That means that the broccoli or carrot or zucchini should be soft—not too crunchy, but not soggy.

Barley was found to have three times more B_{12}. Organically grown foods also have been found to have lower moisture content than those grown conventionally, which could mean that the nutrients in organic foods might not break down as quickly during storage.

But the question of whether organically grown foods have higher nutrient levels than conventionally grown plants has been debated by scientists for decades. They've been unable to reach a clear conclusion on the issue because hard-to-control variables such as

Avoid the thaw. If you buy frozen vegetables, don't let them thaw before cooking them. Freezing the food weakens the cells walls, and that allows nutrients to escape during thawing. Just place the still-frozen vegetables in the microwave, adding only a little bit of water.

Soak the spinach. Before cooking your spinach, let it soak in water for a few minutes. This removes the oxalates that bind with calcium, iron, and other minerals, whisking them out of your body before they can do much good.

Scrub in. Of course, while it's always a good idea to wash produce before you cook it, think twice about peeling edible skins. Carrots and potatoes, for example, are two vegetables that benefit from scrubbing rather than scraping. That's because their skins are richer in minerals than the rest of the vegetable.

Buy small. If you prefer the taste of fresh fruits and vegetables to canned or frozen, cut down the time the produce will need to stay in the refrigerator. Wilting and brown spots are signs of oxidation, which means that the nutrients are slowly leaving the food. Refrigeration will increase the time that fruits and vegetables stay fresh, but only by a day or so.

pesticide residue, but what's done with the plant after harvesting is what can really make the difference between a limp stalk of broccoli that has lost many of its nutrients and a crisp stalk that's rich in vitamins and minerals.

Getting Fresh

Pop quiz: Which of these has the most nutrients?

a. canned vegetables
b. frozen vegetables
c. fresh vegetables

It has to be c. A no-brainer, right? Wrong.

"We did a comparison of the data that are out there, including what's on the cans and packages, and we found that vitamin content is comparable regardless of how you get your vegetables and fruits," says Dr. Barbara Klein of the University of Illinois.

Supermarket fresh translates to produce that is about two weeks old, Dr. Klein says. "So you do just as well using a processed product that has been canned or frozen within hours of being picked," she adds.

For instance, vitamin C in the form of ascorbic acid is an extremely unstable compound. A just-picked orange has about 70 milligrams of vitamin C (nearly 117 percent of the Daily Value). But cook that orange or store it at room temperature and the orange rapidly loses high amounts of its number one nutrient. In fact, orange juice concentrate made immediately after an orange is picked may have more vitamin C than an orange that has traveled from Florida to Idaho in a nonrefrigerated truck.

So it all comes down to this: It doesn't make much difference if you choose fresh, frozen, or canned produce—as long as you eat your fruits and vegetables.

climate and crop variety make it difficult to accurately compare the two farming practices.

But it still may be worth spending a few extra cents to buy organic fruits and vegetables. The USDA recognized more than a decade ago that organic produce contains lower levels of pesticide residue and nitrates. Organic farming is also better for the environment, as it conserves natural resources and cuts down on air, water, and soil pollution.

So how a plant is grown may help determine its nutrient density and its level of

How Vitamin Pills Are Made

From Tons of Raw Materials to a Tablet

Start with a half-ton each of calcium, phosphorus, and magnesium. Mix them with about two tons' worth of 14 or 15 other vitamins and minerals. Divide the whole shebang into a million or so servings, each about ½ inch long and ¼ inch wide. And keep each serving fresh and healthy for three years. That's the challenge vitamin tablet makers face each day.

"It's not easy," says Barry Cason, manager of research and development for Perrigo Company's vitamin and mineral supplement manufacturing facility in Greenville, South Carolina. "And yes, it does involve getting truckloads of vitamins and minerals and finding a way to squish them down into a tablet." Perrigo, is one of the largest private-label nutritional supplement manufacturers. Its products are similar to Centrum, Theragran-M, and One-a-Day. But Perrigo sells them to drugstores, for example, who then put their own names on the formulations.

A supplement manufacturer's first step is to research raw materials. "We have to learn what forms the nutrients are available in, and what each one's price and effectiveness is," says Cason. Calcium carbonate, for example, can come from oyster shells from the ocean or mined limestone purified for humans as well as other sources.

Supplement sources come from all around the world, but there are only a

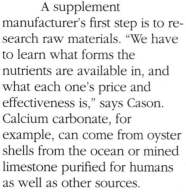

handful of raw material suppliers. And most are used by both the pharmaceutical and food industries. So the thiamin in your vitamin supplement may well come from the same place as the thiamin in your Wonder bread.

Putting It to the Test

After doing research on each source, Cason and his team begin to assemble very small experimental batches of their formulations. "We have to see what will happen to the formulations at various humidities and temperatures," Cason says. "We examine the supplement's reaction at one-, two-, and three-month intervals and extrapolate those findings out to one-year, two-year, and three-year findings." Researchers look for physical and chemical changes as well as potential problems with dissolution.

Dissolution is how the supplement divides into nutrient parts that the body can absorb. In general, vitamins are absorbed in the upper part of the intestine, and minerals mostly in the lower intestine. Water-soluble vitamins are absorbed quickly, while fat-soluble vitamins take longer.

Vitamin manufacturers also sample their products throughout the real shelf-life period at 3, 6, 12, 18, 24, and 36 months, says Cason. Eventually, a performance trial goes to the pilot stage of manufacturing.

One of the greatest challenges for a supplement manufacturer is figuring out how to guarantee that each tablet will deliver its promised amount of every ingredient. Since the master blend of a supplement can weigh a couple of tons, a manufacturer must evenly distribute each ingredient throughout the master blend of a supplement. For instance, if a multivitamin/mineral supplement label claims to have a certain amount of calcium, then controls must be in place to assure that the amount of calcium in the tablet falls within a specified range prescribed by regulation.

"We have to deal with a tremendous amount of weight variations," Cason says. "For example, 162 milligrams of calcium might have to be in the same tablet with 2 milligrams of copper, 400 international units of vitamin D, and 150 micrograms of boron, among 20 other ingredients."

Perrigo, and most other manufacturers, use a specially designed, "twin-shell" blender to mix their nutrients. "It's two huge cylinders that form a V," explains Cason. "Each cylinder spins or tumbles the ingredients. It's almost a kneading action that continuously halves and remixes the dry blend of ingredients, keeping everything evenly distributed."

One process that assists in the blending is called geometric dilution. "There's a sequence to the addition of ingredients," Cason says. "Some of the lighter ingredients are preblended, and we graduate up to heavier ingredients."

Holding It Together

Once the ingredients are mixed together, the trick is to get them to stay together. "A tablet filled with so many ingredients wants to do a lot of things except stay together," says Cason. "It wants to split or fall apart or break up. Or it wants to get so hard that it won't dissolve properly."

A multivitamin/mineral tablet has more than just its active ingredients. It's also filled with excipients, or nonactive ingredients. Each formulation requires a variety of additives to make the nutrients bind together and dissolve properly. Vitamin and mineral supplements come in tablets, liquids, soft gels, and two-piece, hard gelatin capsules. "Tablets are not

only the most popular form for supplements but also the most cost-effective formulation to make," Cason says.

Finally, thousands of tablets are dropped into thousands of bottles and sent to thousands of cities throughout the country. "And we start all over again," says Cason. "New research is always being published, and people want to try different nutrients, like more vitamin E and more antioxidants. Me? I try them all."

Tuning In for Good Health

Most consumers get their information about nutrition from television, but only 17 percent say that they find that information valuable, according to "Nutrition Trends Survey 1995," a study conducted by the American Dietetic Association.

Why? Because one study seems to come to one conclusion and then, a week later, another one contradicts the first report. And let's not forget that the evidence is often "not conclusive."

"The media rarely gives you the bigger picture," says Bonnie Liebman of the Center for Science in the Public Interest. "They say a new study came out with one finding, but they don't tell you that 20 other studies found no link between a vitamin and a disease."

Here are some questions to ask if you want to figure out whether a study is relevant to your life: How much of one vitamin or mineral was studied? Did the researchers look at vitamin and mineral amounts that are found in the diet or in supplements? Once you know the number, compare it to the amount found in your supplement. Also, if you know the amount, try to find out how much of it is found in food. If 500 milligrams of mineral X seems to make a difference in an illness, is there a way to get that solely from food?

Picking the Right Multivitamin for You

The Right Stuff—At the Right Price

One in three American men take multivitamin/mineral supplements. The question is, How can a guy be sure that *he's* not being taken?

Well, first, turn the bottle around and read the fine print. "Don't rely on the opinion of the manufacturer to decide if a supplement is right for you," says Bonnie Liebman of the Center for Science in the Public Interest. "Just because a supplement is labeled 'Men's Formula' doesn't mean that it's exactly what you need to balance out your diet. Special formulas are usually just a marketing gimmick."

It's what's inside the bottle that counts. Don't just look down the right-hand side of the label to see if every nutrient weighs in at 100 percent of the Daily Value. You'll never find 100 percent of every vitamin and mineral in one supplement because with some minerals (calcium, magnesium, phosphorous, and potassium), getting 100 percent of the Daily Value into a single pill would make it too big to swallow.

Plus, you don't need 100 percent of every vitamin and mineral in a pill. What you need to do, dietitians say, is to look for a supplement that at least contains the nutrients usually lacking in the average American man's diet. Those include:

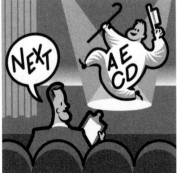

- Vitamin A. Some labels note how much of the supplement's vitamin A comes from beta-carotene (which your body converts into vitamin A). You want 100 percent of the Daily Value, which equals 5,000 international units (IU), with most or all of it coming from beta-carotene. "Most companies mix pre-formed vitamin A with beta-carotene," says Holly McCord, R.D., nutrition editor for *Prevention* magazine. "Either way, there's no reason to go above the Daily Value in a multivitamin/mineral supplement."
- Folic acid. Look for a Daily Value of 100 percent, or 400 micrograms. It's difficult to get this amount in your diet without a lot of planning, so supplementation is a smart move. Some processed foods, mostly bread, will be enriched with folic acid beginning in 1998. That should help, but a supplement with folic acid will still be a good bet.
- Zinc and copper. Get 100 percent of the Daily Value for both of these minerals in a supplement. Keeping them in balance ensures that one won't block absorption of the other.
- Magnesium. You won't find 100 percent of this mineral in a multivitamin/mineral supplement because it would be too big to swallow. Instead, aim to get about 25 percent of the Daily Value, or 100 milligrams, McCord says.
- Chromium. A Daily Value for chromium was only set in 1996 at 120 micrograms, so it may not yet be listed on labels as a percentage of Daily Value. Look for 50 to 200 micrograms, which is in the safe and adequate range.

Buyer Beware

Here are some other key things to look for when you're considering a supplement.

Check the expiration date.

Supplements have a shelf life of about three years, and there's a good chance that you'll happen upon a bargain that offers you 100 tablets with an extra 60 thrown in. That's a five-month supply of vitamins and minerals. Check the date on that package. If it expires soon, it's not worth the money.

Forget about being Mr. Natural. Vitamins and minerals that boast of their "natural" ingredients are usually just money-wasters, Liebman says. In most cases, your body doesn't distinguish between a synthetic vitamin and a natural one.

Form an opinion. Ask yourself, "What form of supplement do I prefer?" If you don't want to swallow tablets, look for a chewable (yes, children's supplements are okay here) or a liquid.

Also, your options will expand if you don't mind taking more than one tablet a day. Many companies offer divided dose supplements to optimize blood levels of nutrients throughout the day.

But be honest: Will you really take more than one tablet a day? If you can't remember where your keys are in the morning or you've had trouble being consistent with vitamin taking in the past, stick with one tablet. Don't make things tough on yourself.

Make sure that the price is right. "There's no reason to spend more than $4 to $5 a month on a multi," Liebman says. "Generally, supplements sold at health food stores cost more than brand names, while generic supplements from large supermarkets or drugstore chains are the cheapest." There is often little difference between the effectiveness of a brand-name and a generic supplement. In fact, they're often made by the same companies. Only the labels change.

"We have to meet the same quality standards as a brand-name company," says Barry Cason of the Perrigo Company, makers of many drugstore and supermarket supplements. "We get the national brand and test it. Then we back it up with independent testing laboratories. In every case our quality meets or exceeds the brand-name product. The only difference is that we don't pay millions of dollars for advertising."

And in reality, that means that *you* don't pay for those advertising costs every time you pop a pill.

But lots of people prefer the security of a brand name, and that's okay, considering the price is only about a dime a day, says Leon Ellenbogen, Ph.D., assistant vice president for Lederle, the makers of Centrum. "Although there are some good generic companies out there, you know exactly what you're buying with a name you recognize. For example, we clinically tested our calcium product, Caltrate, in humans to be certain it's well-absorbed."

Can the iron. There should be something missing from your multivitamin/mineral supplement: iron. "Men don't need added iron," Liebman says. So make sure you choose one without it.

Bringing It All Back Home

Okay, you've made your choice. Here's what to do: Put the bottle somewhere obvious so that you'll remember to take the little buggers. Sure, it's better to store them in a kitchen cabinet, where it's dark and dry, as opposed to the bathroom shelf, where it's humid, but do what's easiest for you.

Or, keep them at work. "Lunch is a great time to take your supplements because drinking them with your morning coffee or tea can actually cut back a bit on mineral absorption," McCord says. "But don't worry if first thing in the morning fits your schedule better. The amount of minerals you might lose is so small that you're still ahead of the game."

And remember that taking vitamins and minerals is like exercise. Sure, you should do it every day. But if you miss a day or two, don't get discouraged. It even happens to the pros.

"I don't remember to take my multi every day," says Liebman. "So don't make yourself crazy."

A Man's Guide to Other Supplements

How to Extend Your Shelf Life

By all means, tune out the crank talk shows and their wild-eyed, Kramer-esque guests who subsist on organic bean sprouts and boiled tofu. But when an herb makes the front page of the venerable *Wall Street Journal*, it's probably time to take notice.

The "other" nutritional supplements have arrived. We're not talking about that alphabet of nutrients that you're beginning to know and love—the ABCs of vitamins. Or their brethren in healing, those magnificent minerals.

Rather, it's that mangy assortment of herbs, oils, and dietary preparations—once relegated to the back of your neighborhood health food store—that are now front and center in the health spotlight. And at your corner drugstore.

The question before the house: Do they work? Answer: A definite maybe, depending on what you choose. "Lots of herbal products definitely have an effect," says William J. Keller, Ph.D., professor and chairman of the department of pharmaceutical sciences at Samford University in Birmingham, Alabama. "They may not have the same striking effect that modern drugs have, but they can be helpful, depending on the condition."

Some supplements, like amino acids, glucosamine sulfate, and hormone replacements, will require more research before we know. But one thing is certain: You're bound to encounter more and

more of them. Here's a guy's guide to what you'll see along the way. If you think one of these might be right for you and your doctor hasn't already left for the country club, see what he thinks. Always check with your doctor before taking any herbal products, especially if taking medication, because there can be harmful interactions, says Dr. Keller.

Amino acids. Used by Arnold Schwarzenegger wanna-bes, amino acids are frequently featured in bodybuilding magazines. While research shows that you need to eat more protein when you're trying to pack on lean body mass, the evidence for amino acids is tougher to come by—if you're already getting adequate protein. Originally used to prevent protein loss in folks recovering from surgery, amino acids are simply protein building blocks such as l-isoleucine, l-leucine, and l-glutamine. Although there are some small studies that show that amino acid supplements help burn fat and build muscle, more needs to be done. There are also some side effects, such as nausea and diarrhea, that you may want to do without.

Brewer's yeast. With a name like that, it has to be good, right? If you're looking for a mother lode of vitamins and minerals in one tablet, brewer's yeast delivers. Most contain thiamin, riboflavin, niacin, pyridoxine, pantothenic acid, biotin, and folic acid, not to mention chromium and selenium. Two studies note that it may also contain chemicals that speed wound healing. And yes, it's the actual stuff that's

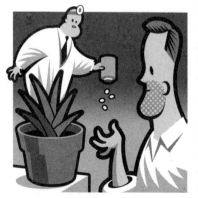

needed to make beer—without the alcohol, of course, says Dr. Keller. And although brewer's yeast is rich in various relatively nontoxic nutrients, follow the label's instructions because dosage can vary widely among products.

Capsaicin. The next time you attempt your Dick Butkus imitation at the company flag football game, you might want to reach for some capsaicin. Applying this red-pepper derivative topically has been found to reduce aches and pains by what might be called the lights-are-on-but-nobody's-home mechanism—simply helping thwart the transmission of pain signals to your brain.

This same principle apparently came in handy during at least one double-blind study of arthritis sufferers with hand pain. Those who rubbed on capsaicin cream for nine weeks had 22 percent less pain than the folks who got placebos (fake pills). You may also see capsaicin in candy, capsule, or cream form to treat mouth sores in cancer patients, belly aches, psoriasis, and even the mysterious burning in the legs and feet of AIDS sufferers. Capsaicin cream is available without a prescription. Make sure to clean your hands thoroughly after you apply capsaicin though: It will burn your eyes and just about anything else that's tender.

DHEA. Forget Ponce de Leon: To enthusiastic supporters, the supplement DHEA (dehydroepiandrosterone) is a fountain of youth that can build muscle, boost memory, and aid immune function. How? Called the mother hormone—or as Saddam Hussein might say, the Mother of All Hormones—DHEA circulates in your body helping produce that manly stuff called testosterone. As you get older, however, your body progressively makes less, leading (Heaven forbid) to aging. Replacing your dwindling DHEA supply by taking a supplement is thought to slow the process—or so supporters say. This sounds logical, but we don't know enough about DHEA yet to say whether it will live up to its claims. DHEA has not been tested in controlled, long-term clinical trials, and it is not regulated for strength and purity in the United States. So you don't know if you are getting DHEA or something else entirely. Anecdotal reports among bodybuilders, even health journalists, do suggest that it may indeed add bulk.

Echinacea. Rhymes with "Glad I met ya." The subject of a front-page *Wall Street Journal* article, echinacea is one of the best-selling herbal remedies on the market. The reason why the cash register is ringing is because regular folks swear it can help ward off a cold and flu—or at least shorten the length and severity. What do doctors say? "Echinacea definitely stimulates the nonspecific immune system," says Dr. Keller. "In other words, it stimulates the cells that eliminate cold viruses and other harmful cells. It's probably one of the most viable herbal treatments around." For a two-fisted, cold-fighting punch, consider taking vitamin C and echinacea. Take echinacea at the first sign of cold or flu symptoms according to package directions, says Dr. Keller. And don't take it for long periods of time, as it could begin to depress your immune system. You won't confuse it with a full-bodied pilsner, however: Echinacea tastes lousy in its most potent form—liquid.

Feverfew. Arthritis and migraine sufferers have turned to this herb in droves for relief. The active ingredient has been identified as parthenolide, but you may not be getting what you expect in pill form. Feverfew supplements are notoriously unreliable in their quality and potency. If you have a green thumb, try growing some yourself and chewing on one or two leaves. Discontinue use immediately if feverfew leaves irritate your mouth.

Fish oil. If you've started walking like former New York Jets Hall of Famer Joe Namath, you may want to think about adding fish oil to your diet. A review of 10 double-blind studies found that folks with arthritis who took 3 to 6 grams of fish oil a day had a modest benefit—without apparent side effects. Not only that, but fish oil figures to be heart-healthy, lowering blood pressure, reducing blood fat levels, and increasing clotting times. One British study showed that heart attack survivors who ate more fish, the best source of fish oil, were 29 percent less likely to die within the next few years than guys who hadn't added fish to their dish. The American Heart Association prefers that you get your fish oil from fish because you're less likely to overdose, which can lead to excessive bleeding, drug interactions, and possibly high cholesterol.

Flaxseed oil. We're just beginning to get the facts on flax, but here's what we know so far: Like fish, it contains omega-6 fatty acids but actually has more omega-3 fatty acids—both considered heart-healthy. It's also one of the best sources of what's called gamma-lineolinic acid, a substance that may help arthritis sufferers. What's more, flax may ease asthma and allergic reactions and boost your immune system. Add the oil to yogurt, or grind up and sprinkle the seeds the next time you bake—it's a grain after all.

Garlic. You know it as the breath smell of doom, but there's a growing body of evidence suggesting that garlic will do more than ruin your chances for a smooch on your first date. In an analysis of several studies—called a metanalysis by the guys in the lab coats—taking dried garlic seemed to be of some benefit for people with mildly elevated blood pressure. The same authors also found that 600 to 900 milligrams of dried garlic a day reduced bad cholesterol and blood fat. They do admit that more trials should be done before wholeheartedly promoting garlic. Available in deodorized form, garlic has also been found to have a mild immune-boosting effect, says Dr. Keller, which might help ward off colds.

Ginger. Not only has ginger been found to reduce motion sickness and upset stomach, but it naturally aids digestion. How well? In one study, 940 milligrams of ginger outperformed 100 milligrams of dimenhydrinate (Dramamine) for motion sickness. And although a study funded by the National Aeronautics and Space Administration didn't find any benefit, 1 gram of ginger helped keep green Navy cadets from turning green when they were exposed to choppy seas.

Ginkgo. Considered a conventional drug in Europe, ginkgo has been shown to improve circulation problems, leading some to use it for conditions ranging from intermittent claudi-cation (slowed blood flow in the legs) to tinnitis (ringing in the ears). You'll also see it in various formulations suggesting improved brain functions, such as boosting short-term memory,

relieving headaches, and even combating vertigo.

If you choose to try ginkgo, make sure that it is a standardized formula. The recommended dosage is a 40-milligram tablet or capsule three times a day, according to Dr. Keller. Ginkgo is generally regarded as safe, but since it affects the body's clotting mechanism, use caution if taking aspirin or anticlotting med-ications. Some people may experience mild side effects, such as restlessness and digestive upset and should discontinue use.

Ginseng. Don't be surprised if you see the cartoon character Dilbert giving this Chinese herb to his boss someday. In a study of 95 British middle managers, those who had a poor diet and took a multivitamin containing 40 mil-ligrams of ginseng reported less anxiety, anger, and confusion and more vigor than those who were given a placebo. Long touted by the Chi-nese as an aphrodisiac, ginseng is thought to be what's called an adaptogen, which means that it's supposed to help you better cope with stress. And that, in turn, may help you perform better sexually, says Dr. Keller. Ginseng has also been used successfully on conditions ranging from diabetes to clogged arteries, conditions that can cause sexual dysfunction. Some side effects of ginseng include insomnia and possibly diarrhea. However, since quality control is extremely difficult to maintain, you may not be getting quality ginseng or any ginseng at all in that supplement.

Glucosamine sulfate. There are lots of reasons to look forward to old age: senior citizen discounts, the right to wear Bermuda shorts, a sudden fascination with Guy Lombardo, and so on. But sadly, you also seem to produce less glucosamine, a substance that helps keep your cartilage strong and rigid. Less glucosamine, then, and before long it's Canasta City: Your cartilage breaks down, causing one form of the familiar joint pain and stiffness known as arthritis. The question is, can swallowing synthetic glucosamine sulfate capsules replace that lost glucosamine and save your joints? By the looks of health food store and drugstore shelves that stock the stuff, you'd think so. There have been several promising small, controlled trials done overseas testing glucosamine sulfate as an effective treatment for arthritis. And although some short-term pain relief was found, studies have yet to determine any long-term benefits. The Arthritis Foundation does not recommend the use of glucosamine sulfate in the treatment of arthritis and cautions that since it is considered a dietary supplement, it is not regulated by the Food and Drug Administration (FDA).

If you choose to take glucosamine sulfate, the dosage is a 500-milligram capsule three times a day, says Dr. Keller. There are virtually no side effects, but some people do complain of nausea.

Goldenseal root. Goldenseal is thought to make a nifty tea for soothing canker sores, chapped lips, and an otherwise sore mouth. It also comes in capsules, but its effects when taken internally are unreliable. Check with your doctor before taking goldenseal internally, as it may increase blood pressure.

Hawthorn. Keep your eye on this herb. Research has shown that hawthorn can help open coronary blood vessels, often lowering blood pressure. Not only that, but hawthorn is thought to "reduce the tendency to angina attacks," according to Varro E. Tyler, Ph.D., in his book *The Honest Herbal*, and even aid the heart after injury from an attack.

If you think that hawthorn may help you, consult a doctor familiar with hawthorn. Don't try to self-diagnose heart problems, says Dr. Keller. They require a doctor's expertise.

Pycnogenol. One of the most recent entrants in the supplement wars, you'll probably be hearing a lot about pycnogenol in the future. Made from the bark of the European coastal pine tree, pycnogenol contains chemicals called bioflavonoids that are thought to protect your cardiovascular system from free-radical damage. Much of the advertising information promoting pycnogenol is based on the tale of a French explorer and his crew who were given pine tea brewed by an Indian. This

tea cured the crew members of scurvy. An interesting bedtime story for the kids, but until some serious studies of pycnogenol's antioxidant qualities are done, stick with reliable and cheaper forms of bioflavonoids, such as citrus fruits, blueberries, tea, onions, and apples. You could also have a reaction if you are allergic to pine.

Saw palmetto. This extract of the saw palmetto berry has been found in some studies to relieve symptoms caused by nonmalignant enlargement of the prostate. In one study of 500 guys suffering from benign prostatic hyperplasia (BPH), 88 percent experienced reduction in their symptoms. Because the active chemicals of saw palmetto are fat-soluble, not water-soluble, drinking a tea made from the berries won't help your prostate. Also, you won't see saw palmetto advertising that it is beneficial for BPH. The FDA has not approved it for sale for BPH in the United States. You may find it, however, in some over-the-counter male potency supplements.

Soy. From hot dogs and burger patties to milk, you're certain to encounter some soy in your travels. And it's not just vegetarians trying to avoid meat who are buying the stuff. A series of studies have found that soybeans contain a chemical called isoflavones that may help prevent heart disease as well prostate and other kinds of cancer. Also, soy products generally contain less saturated fat than meat—another source of cardiovascular problems. If you don't mind trading some taste for potential health benefits, you might give it a try, says Dr. Keller.

Valerian. Better than 2 hours of The Weather Channel, valerian has long been known for its mild tranquilizing effect. As a result, it's often recommended in Germany as a sleep aid or for restlessness. "It doesn't have the same potency as a prescription sleep aid, but it will definitely make you drowsy," Dr. Keller says. Be sure to follow label instructions and cautions. Check with your doctor before taking valerian if you are taking central nervous system depressants such as diazepam (Valium), and as with any product that causes drowsiness, don't operate a car or heavy machinery.

A Guy's Guide to Sports and Energy Bars

Eating on the Run

We won't kid you, men: Cushioned insoles are probably easier to chew than many sports and energy bars on the market today. And taste? Suffice it to say that if your mom served similar-tasting meals when you were a kid, there's a good chance that we're going to see your mug on America's Most Wanted. One grizzled runner, disgusted after sampling several different brands, referred to the lot as the "Spam of the 1990s"—clearly a not-so-flattering reference to that much-maligned meat product.

But when it comes to convenience, portability, caloric density, and nutrient content, sports and energy bars deserve a second look. For one thing, many deliver at least half the vitamins and minerals a guy needs in a day—some even more. Not only that, but if you wanted a comparable nonanimal high-protein source that's as low in fat, you'd have to find the time to cook up a huge plate of rice and beans—or find someone to do it for you—and then find the time and tools to sit down and eat it. Even folks who are lactose-intolerant will find something here. Many manufacturers use lactose- and dairy-free proteins. And frankly, when it comes to taste, even the most finicky agree: A few are surprisingly good.

"There are so many reasons why sports bars make sense for busy and active people," says Kristine Clark, R.D., Ph.D., director of sports nutrition at the Pennsylvania

State Center for Sports Medicine at Pennsylvania State University in University Park. "I use them, my clients use them, and I feel better and better about recommending them. It's a very competitive product now."

You don't need a stopwatch to figure out why sports and energy bars win with athletes on the go or who are about to compete, says Dr. Clark. "They need nonperishable stuff that can be carried in a gym bag or golf bag or on an airplane, and these bars fit the bill," she says.

Okay, so you don't have to lug a refrigerator or cooler along with you when you have a sports bar handy. That's why they made healthy choices at fast-food restaurants, right? "A lot of athletes don't want to eat much solid food even 3 to 4 hours before an event. It may be somewhat psychological, but they don't like going into an event feeling like their gut is full. That's where a compact, strong caloric contribution from a small package is not just handy but valuable," says Dr. Clark.

Desk jockeys can also benefit. Remember all those times that you have been forced to forage at the candy machine after missing lunch? And guys who aren't thrilled with the prospect of eggs—or anything else at 7:00 A.M.—are finding that a sports or energy bar does the trick, says Susan Kundrat, R.D., a sports nutritionist and coordinator of the SportWell Center at University of Illinois in Champaign. "Obviously, a real food source is always better, but it's so important to eat something in the morning that I recommend energy bars to guys who won't eat anything else," she says.

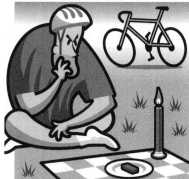

But it's not enough to grab any old bar off the shelf. Here's how to make the best of a sports bar.

Cram those carbs. If you're eating a sports bar right before training or an athletic event, it's probably best to stick with one high in carbohydrates and low in protein, fat, and fiber. Why? These normally healthy ingredients slow digestion, withholding the energy boost you need. Instead, says Dr. Clark, look for one made primarily from glucose, sucrose, or fructose. Perhaps the best pre-event bars are those with four to five times the number of carbohydrates as proteins or fat.

Beat the clock. Most sports bar manufacturers recommend eating their product no later than 30 minutes before training or competition, but Dr. Clark says that 2 to 3 hours may be even better. "It's going to sustain your energy level and keep you feeling relatively satiated during your event," she says. The longer the time before the event, the more protein, fiber, and fat your bar can have, she says. In fact, one of the bars on the market that contains 40 percent carbohydrates, 30 percent protein, and 30 percent fat would be ideal for that kind of situation, she says.

Wash it down with water. You won't need a reminder to have a tall glass of water on hand when you're trying to chew a sports or energy bar, but by then it could be too late. And not just because nearly all of these things are tough to swallow: "They're such tremendous sources of concentrated energy, you actually run the risk of dehydration or stomach cramping if you don't get enough fluids," Kundrat says. A few extra 8-ounce glasses of water should be enough to help you choke one down and keep you from becoming dehydrated.

Balance it with a banana. A sports bar gobbled on the way to work doesn't exactly qualify as a hearty breakfast. But add a bagel or a piece of fruit like a banana and you're getting between 300 and 400 calories—a strong way to start your morning. "The way I see it, you should have about a third of your daily calories before noon, but it doesn't have to be in one fell swoop," says Dr. Clark. "If you don't like to eat breakfast at 7:00 A.M., you can have something like this at 9:00 A.M., some more at 10:00, and more at 11:00. This type of morning meal fits in

Passing the Bar

If sports and energy bars are too chalky—or costly—for you to swallow, have an old-fashioned "sports bar," like a granola or fig bar, or even a banana. You can get just as much energy from these foods—all of which cost pennies per serving—as from a $2 to $3 sports bar. Here's what you get, according to Nancy Clark, R.D., author of *Nancy Clark's Sports Nutrition Guidebook*.

Bar	Calories	Carbohydrate (g.)	Protein (g.)	Fat (g.)
Granola Bar	109	16	2	4
Fig Bar	200	42	2	3
Banana	105	27	1	0.6

nicely with the sensible and healthy recommendation that you spread your calories out."

Do higher protein post-event. If you're interested in a post-event or postworkout snack, and there's no way to get your hands on some real food, make sure that your bar is high in protein—especially if you're a vegetarian, bodybuilder, or power athlete. "Generally, you need 1 to 1.2 grams of protein per kilogram of body weight daily," says Dr. Clark. "Some guys who are training super hard may need as much as 2.4 grams of protein per kilogram a day." For a moderately active, 180-pound guy, that's about 90 grams of protein a day—roughly two cans of water-packed tuna.

Look for one that's fat-friendly. Be aware that some bars, while relatively low in fat, may contain oils that have been altered so that they have a longer shelf life. The result is that more research needs to be done, but these "fractionalized" or "hydrogenated" oils may be less heart-healthy. "If you're really concerned about this issue, avoid products made with hydrogenated oil completely or make sure that the oils that have been hydrogenated are monounsaturated fats such as peanut oil, olive oil, canola oil, or rapeseed oil," says Dr. Clark.

The Sports and Energy Bar Taste Challenge

When we decided to taste-test sports/energy bars, we assembled some of the toughest judges imaginable: grizzled health journalists and editors who have sampled nearly every so-called healthy food that has hit the market. The results weren't pretty: They complained a lot and drank enough to water to drown a gym rat. But when the plates were cleaned, there was no denying it: Several bars emerged as clear winners in our first-ever sports and energy bar taste-off. Below are details of the five top finishers.

Bar	Size (oz.)	Calories	Protein (g.)	Fat (g.)	Carbo-hydrates (sugar), g.	Vitamin A (% of Daily Value)	Vitamin B$_{12}$ (% of Daily Value)	Vitamin C (% of Daily Value)
Clif Bar: The Natural Energy Bar (Peanut Butter)	2.4	250	10	4	45 (10)	0	Not available	0
PR Bar Ironman Triathlon Nutrition Bar (Yogurt Berry)	2	230	16	8	24 (16)	50	50	50
Tiger's Milk (Peanut Butter and Honey)	1.25	150	5	5	20 (13)	15	25	10
Pure Protein Meal Replacement Sports Bar (Peanut Butter)	2.8	280	33	7	9 (6)	100	100	100
Balance: The Complete Nutritional Food Bar (Honey Peanut)	1.76	190	15	6	22 (17)	50	30	200

In making their decisions, the judges were encouraged to consider such factors as appearance, flavor, chewability, and aftertaste. No nutritional or ingredient information was provided at the time of the test, lest it sway their taste buds. One note: The Daily Values for each of these bars are based on a 2,000-calorie diet, which is below the needs for the typical active adult male. The rating scale was from 1 (awful, I'd rather eat tree bark) to 10 (tasty, I'd share it with my pals).

Vitamin E (% of Daily Value)	Magnesium (% of Daily Value)	Zinc (% of Daily Value)	First six ingredients	Taste rating	Judge's comment
Not available	Not available	Not available	Rolled oats, FruitSource (whole rice syrup, grape juice concentrate), brown rice syrup, rice crisp, natural peanut butter, brown rice protein	6.25	"Delightful. If this were softer, I could spread it on some bread and eat it with jelly. Hearty peanut butter flavor."
50	50	50	Special Ironman protein (consisting of soy protein isolate, soybeans, whey protein concentrate, and calcium sodium caseinate), high-fructose corn syrup, peanut butter, sucrose, glycerine, fractionated palm kernel oil	5.5	"Yum! Tasty vanilla icing."
Not available	25	Not available	Carob coating (brown sugar, partially hydrogenated vegetable oils [cottonseed, soybean], whey powder, carob powder, soy lecithin), peanut butter (peanuts, dextrose, hydrogenated vegetable oils [rapeseed, cottonseed, soybean], salt), brown sugar, honey, corn syrup, brown rice flour	5.4	"Close to an actual candy bar."
Not available	25	100	Ionic whey protein, calcium caseinate, chocolate coating (beet sugar, fractionated canola oil, cocoa powder, nonfat dry milk, lecithin), peanut flour, natural flavors, glycerine	4.9	"Looks and tastes like Snicker's bar in disguise. Aftertaste spoils the fun."
200	10	35	Protein blend (soy protein isolate, calcium caseinate, toasted soybeans, whey protein concentrate, whey), high-fructose corn syrup, honey, high-maltose corn syrup, sugar, palm and palm kernel oils	4.5	"Much better than its mocha-flavored cousin."

Designing a Smart Supplementing Strategy

Good Health Insurance for Life

In some ways, figuring out your vitamin and mineral supplementation program is like creating an investment portfolio. The shrewd man starts in his early twenties with a multivitamin/mineral supplement to round out his diet, providing protection against minor setbacks such as skipping meals, catching a cold, or working late for several nights in a row. But just as your financial needs grow larger and more complex as you age—buying a house, sending kids to college, retirement—so do your nutritional needs. After a certain age, one tablet just won't be enough.

The shrewd man in his forties begins to understand the need to diversify his nutritional portfolio, targeting several specific areas of health concerns. Part of his plan is simply guarding against the natural erosion that accompanies aging. But now he can also hedge his bets against the prime men killers—heart disease and cancer, chief among them.

Some men will want to find a single magic pill to cover all the bases—some little miracle that will guarantee a cancer-free, high-energy, high-sex, stress-free life. Unfortunately, vitamin and mineral supplements can't give you that, although, like you, we wish they could.

In fact, the real secret to nutritional health lies in casting your net wide. For instance, when researchers gave a multivitamin/mineral supplement to a small group of elderly people with good nutritional habits, they found that those who took the supplement had stronger immune systems than those who didn't. However, the researchers didn't look for one secret ingredient in the supplements. Nor did they assume that this supplement was the one supplement that could prolong life. Instead they concluded that each person benefited in his or her own way from the wide variety of nutrients available in the supplement.

In fact, doctors haven't yet come to the conclusion that supplement takers live longer. It's almost impossible to attribute longevity to supplements alone. However, supplement users tend to have healthier diets and lifestyles than those who don't take supplements.

The Dynamic Duo

The key is to supplement knowledgeably. The first step is to identify your own particular needs and risks. You could be getting the Daily Values for all of the major vitamins and minerals but still not be getting what you need for optimal performance.

"The Daily Values represent the minimum wage of nutrients," says Alexander Schauss, Ph.D., director of the life sciences division of the American Institute for Biosocial Research in Tacoma, Washington, and author of *Minerals, Trace Elements, and Human Health*. "They offer little hope of significantly improving the quality of your life."

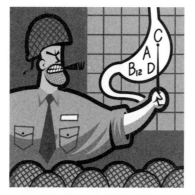

Similarly, a multivitamin/mineral supplement straight from your drugstore represents the minimum wage of supplementation. Don't get us wrong: They're a great, inexpensive tool for many people. But if you're looking to live at a more challenging level, we're willing to bet that you'd like a supplementation program specifically geared to your own lifestyle and goals.

When it comes to vitamins, many experts agree that the true powerhouses are C and E. Almost every guy should be supplementing with these for optimal health.

Start with vitamin C. The Daily Value for vitamin C is 60 milligrams, which seems quite low in the face of recent research. And, although one orange will give you the daily minimum, only about half of all Americans eat fruit every day. At the same time, research has shown that we seem to benefit from dosages at much higher levels than 60 milligrams. This is especially true for smokers, people who live in cities, and those who exercise a lot, says Dr. Schauss.

"Smokers and other people whose lungs take a beating should get a minimum of 200 milligrams a day of vitamin C and 100 international units (IU) of vitamin E," says Dr. Alan Gaby of Bastyr University. "Taking a supplement of 250 to 500 milligrams of vitamin C a day is safe for just about everyone. I recommend vitamin C supplementation to nearly all my patients." Remember, though, that doses of 1,200 milligrams or higher sometimes cause intestinal problems (specifically diarrhea), so there's no need to go overboard unless there is a medical reason for the higher dose.

It isn't that difficult, actually, to eat a lot of vitamin C every day. Down a big glass of orange juice with breakfast and you'll get about 150 milligrams. Eat some red bell peppers and some broccoli at lunch and you'll hit the 250-milligram mark.

Give yourself an E for effort. Two words: heart disease. If you wanted to stick strictly with food products for your vitamin E, you'd wind up getting a lot of excess fat because the richest sources of vitamin E are oils: hazelnut, sunflower, almond, and

---

A Supplementation Self-Test

Here is a list of questions developed by Dr. Alexander Schauss of the American Institute for Biosocial Research to identify people who could most benefit from increasing their intakes of certain nutrients:

- Are you at high risk due to family history or lifestyle for illnesses such as cancer, cardiovascular disease, or diabetes?
- Do you exercise at least three times a week?
- Are you under a lot of stress?
- Do you have skin problems?
- Do you want to strengthen your immune system?
- Do you frequently drink alcohol?
- Do you smoke or are you exposed to secondhand smoke at home or work?
- Do you live in an area with high pollution rates?
- Did a diet or nutritional analysis indicate a deficiency of any nutrients?
- Do you have a diagnosed degenerative disease?
- Do you drink more than 3 cups of coffee or 5 to 6 cups of tea (all types) a day?
- Are you over 50?

If you answer yes to at least one of these questions, you may need additional vitamin or mineral supplementation. Discuss with your doctor which vitamins and minerals could be helpful to you and your health, and always check with your doctor before supplementing, says Dr. Schauss.

---

cottonseed. "You can't eat enough vitamin E to get enough of the heart-protective effects," Dr. Gaby says. "You'd have to drink cups of unprocessed sunflower oil, which would be both disgusting and fattening." The solution? Supplementation.

There's lots of evidence, says Dr. Gaby, that men who take vitamin E have lower heart disease risk. The Daily Value is 30 IU, but studies have suggested supplementing in amounts of 100 to 400 IU. Many popular multivitamin/mineral supplements have 30 IU of vitamin E, which wouldn't be enough to see a particular effect against heart disease. Instead, consider taking a vitamin E supplement or an antioxidant supplement that includes both vitamins C and E, says Dr. Gaby.

Key Minerals for Men

Even the most hardy man of the soil probably could use a little help when it comes to getting the minerals he needs. Here are some important minerals for a supplementation plan, according to Dr. Gaby.

Mine extra magnesium. The average American man doesn't get enough of this mineral from food. While it is usually included in multivitamin/mineral supplements, magnesium is a big, bulky mineral. It's hard to get 100 percent of the Daily Value (let alone anything higher) into a tablet filled with other nutrients. Centrum, for example, has just 25 percent of the Daily Value, or 100 milligrams.

Consider calcium. Another mineral that may be difficult to consume enough of in a normal diet is calcium—unless you're drinking three glasses of milk a day or the equivalent. Because men drink more milk than women and don't see problems with osteoporosis until much later in life, they don't worry about this mineral as much as they should. However, it's the milk you drink in your twenties and thirties that will save your spine in your seventies and eighties.

Add zinc. Extra zinc also is recommended. Fortunately, zinc, magnesium, and calcium are often grouped together in a single supplement. The problem is that if you take extra zinc, you should also be sure that your multivitamin/mineral supplement contains at least the Daily Value for copper, since excess zinc intake can cause copper deficiency.

"Look for 200 to 400 milligrams of magnesium, 400 to 800 milligrams of calcium, 15 milligrams of zinc, and 2 milligrams of copper in a supplement," Dr. Gaby recommends.

Ask Questions

If you have your own set of aches and pains, chances are good that nutrition and possibly supplementation can help you there, too. Many illnesses and symptoms can be relieved, and some even cured, with nutritional therapy.

"There's circumstantial evidence that, for example, riboflavin can prevent migraines and niacin or niacinamide can treat osteoarthritis," Dr. Gaby says. "But, in these examples, nutrition is becoming a prescription. It's important to do your research and, if possible, find a doctor who will work with you on using vitamins and minerals as medication or therapy. Large doses of niacinamide, doses in the 2,000- to 3,000-milligram range that is used to treat osteoarthritis, can stress and damage the liver."

You may be reading this as an energetic, overeating 25-year-old; a hard-working, overextended 40-year-old; or even a trying-to-keep-young 65-year-old. But each of you should remember that nutritional needs vary according to your stage of life. As you age, your nutritional needs will change. And you should stay in touch with those changes and respond appropriately.

The Daily Values group everyone over the age of 51 into one category, but we live much longer than that now. Likewise, studies have shown that while people decrease the amount of food they eat as they get older, they don't increase their micronutrients. In fact, for generations physicians have considered aging and its symptoms inevitable, but researchers have found specific lifestyle and diet-related changes that contribute to the diseases and problems of the elderly. From weight gain to disease, many problems of aging are related to nutrition.

In fact, part of aging is the decline of many nutrient and hormone levels in the body. For instance, chromium supplies simply deplete as we age. You can alter this easily with supplements. Most multivitamin/mineral supplements contain the minimum recommended amount of chromium. "The supplement will help replenish depleted stores," Dr. Gaby says.

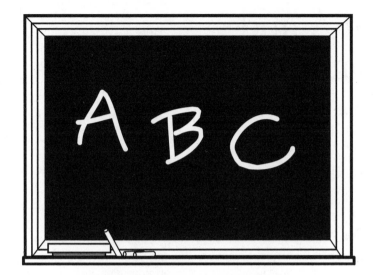

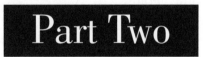
Part Two

Know Your ABCs

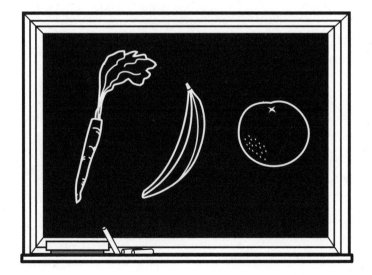

Vitamin A and Beta-Carotene

• **Where You Get It:** Liver and carrots (richest sources); dark green, leafy vegetables (spinach, collard and mustard greens); yellow vegetables (squash, pumpkins, sweet potatoes); yellow fruits (peaches, apricots).

• **What It Does for You:** Keeps your eyes healthy; prevents night blindness; is essential for body growth and normal tooth development; protects and maintains linings of the throat and respiratory, digestive, and urinary systems; helps with protein and glycogen synthesis.

• **What a Man Needs:** Daily Value of 5,000 international units (IU).

• **Cautions:** Too little can cause night blindness; stunt growth in children; promote tooth pitting and decay; create rough, dry, scaly skin; and cause reproductive disorders. Taking more than 50,000 IU per day over a long period of time can lead to headaches, blurred vision, loss of hair, dry skin (with flaking and itching), drowsiness, diarrhea, nausea, and enlargement of the liver and spleen. Acute toxicity, and even death, may occur in massive doses of 2,000,000 to 5,000,000 IU daily.

Vitamin A is probably the most important vitamin to your body. That certainly qualifies it as interesting. But more astounding is this: You need vitamin A to live but can't make it on your own, so you eat plants. And here's the rub: Plants don't have any vitamin A either.

Confused?

Don't be. This little chemical conundrum is what makes vitamin A so exciting—and so important. Read on to learn why you, like Arthur Fonzarelli in *Happy Days*, should also be saying, "Aaaaaaaaaay."

Three Blind Mice

Every living animal, including man, the wildest animal of all, needs vitamin A to live. Vitamin A, as a scientist would say, is the product of animal metabolism, which means that your body—and the body of every species of mammal, bird, and fish—manufactures vitamin A internally through the physiology of life and living.

Most of the vitamin A you need comes from the food you eat, particularly plants. Yet, plants themselves don't have any vitamin A. Their chemical counterpart is a similar substance called carotene, a yellow-colored, fat-soluble substance that gives the characteristic yellow-orange color to carrots. (Carotene got its name because it was first isolated from carrots more than 100 years ago.) As a result, the ultimate source of man's vitamin A comes from carotene synthesized by plants. Our bodies, and the bodies of other animals, take the carotene—also called a vitamin A precursor—and, through the wonders of our metabolic chemistry sets, turn it into vitamin A. In other words, plants have the ingredients for vitamin A, but it's your body that mixes the batter.

"To put it another way, vitamin A really isn't a true vitamin at all. Your body can make it from carotene," says Michael Janson, M.D., president of the American Preventive Medicine Association and director of the Center for Preventive Medicine in Barnstable, Massachusetts, and author of *The Vitamin Revolution in Health Care.*

As for the history of vitamin A, it is—like

a carrot—long and colorful, in part, because vitamin A is older than Methuselah. Early remedies using vitamin A surfaced in ancient China, where the Chinese made vitamin A–rich concoctions to treat night blindness. Later, in Greece, Hippocrates, the father of modern medicine, did pretty much the same when he prescribed various preparations of liver to treat the same malady because liver, too, is rich in vitamin A. (Night blindness, or nyctalopia, is a condition in which your eyes lose their ability to adequately adjust to dim light.)

Such antiquated home remedies prospered through the ages but did little to clarify vitamin A's role as a chemical. That type of specific research didn't yield appreciable results until the early 1900s.

Definitive findings on vitamin A came in 1913, when four scientists operating independently in two labs discovered vitamin A by demonstrating that there was an essential substance in fatty foods. Elmer V. McCollum and Marguerite Davis of the University of Wisconsin discovered vitamin A in butter fat and egg yolks, while Thomas B. Osborne and Lafayette B. Mendel of the Connecticut Experiment Station discovered it in cod-liver oil. In those two landmark experiments, the four scientists found that the absence of vitamin A caused eye problems in animals. Two years later, McCollum and Davis fine-tuned their research to directly link vitamin A deficiency with night blindness, thus answering for good the real reason that Hippocrates was such a liver fan.

Following this pioneering work, vitamin A attracted the attention of scientists all over the world within two short decades. In 1920, an English scientist proposed the official "vitamin A" name. It was previously called fat-soluble A. Other scientists discovered similar substances in other foods, like sweet potatoes and corn.

A or B-C?

When it comes to taking supplements, most experts agree that you're better off taking them to round out a healthy, nutritious diet—not to take the place of a healthy, nutritious diet. That is, except when it comes to vitamin A and beta-carotene.

Enormous amounts of vitamin A can be toxic. Too much beta-carotene, while not toxic, can turn your skin orange. The question is, if you want extra A, what do you do?

For starters, talk to your dietitian or physician. After that, consider taking beta-carotene supplements in addition to vitamin A, says Dr. Michael Janson of the American Preventive Medicine Association and the Center for Preventive Medicine. That's because beta-carotene is converted into vitamin A by your body at its leisure.

Beta-carotene is nontoxic, so for higher levels of intake, stick to that. But look carefully at labels that say vitamin A *with* beta-carotene. If the label doesn't specify, you can't be sure how much of each you're getting.

These substances would later be called carotene.

Despite these exciting findings, the true defining moment for vitamin A—and a defining moment in the history of vitamins and nutrition in general—came in 1931, when a Swiss researcher isolated the active substance in halibut-liver oil and analyzed it for its chemical content. His work resulted in vitamin A being the first vitamin ever to have its chemical structure decoded. For this, researcher Paul Karrar received the Nobel prize.

A Recipe for Confusion

In comparison to that larval state of research in the early twentieth century, science today has much to say about vitamin A and carotene. Today, for example, the relationship between vitamin A and the carotenes is clear. The problem, however, is that the details are clear to scientists but not necessarily to laymen, says Maye Musk, R.D., an international nutrition consultant, speaker, and author of *Feel Fantastic.*

"Most people aren't really sure about vitamin A and carotene or beta-carotene, and rightly so," Musk says. "More than 600 carotenoids are found in nature, and 50 of them have the potential for vitamin A activity. When you say that—and throw in the fact that beta-carotene can be found in orange fruits and vegetables, like mangoes and carrots, *and* in green, leafy vegetables, like broccoli, *and* that vitamin A is found in animal products—you have a recipe for confusion."

Here's the scoop: Vitamin A is a misleading name. It's not truly one substance. There are, in fact, several forms of vitamin A, each with varying degrees of potency. The two main types of vitamin A are retinol and dehydroretinol. Then there are the carotenes. These are the precursors to vitamin A, the substances found in fruits and vegetables. Carotenes help us make vitamin A through metabolism.

The four most powerful carotenes vitamin A–wise are called alpha-carotene, beta-carotene, gamma-carotene, and cryptoxanthine, which is a carotene found in corn. Of these four heavy-hitting carotenes, beta-carotene has the highest potential to create vitamin A, alone providing about two-thirds of the vitamin A that your body needs to survive. That's precisely why it gets all the attention when talk turns to vitamin A.

"These carotenes give some of those fruits and vegetables their characteristic colors," Musk says. "But just because you don't see yellow or orange doesn't mean they're not present. In other foods, like broccoli, for example, the carotene is there. It's just masked by chlorophyll, the substance that gives plants their green color."

As for its utility, vitamin A serves the body in several important ways. In addition to its well-known role in maintaining healthy vision and in preventing blindness and night blindness, vitamin A does the following:

- Spurs overall growth. In addition to helping growth at the cellular level, vitamin A is indirectly responsible for your sense of taste. Without enough vitamin A, the cells that make up your taste buds dry out, or keratinize, because there isn't enough vitamin A to help those cells properly develop. Because your taste buds are on the fritz, you lose your sense of taste and thus your appetite and ability to grow.
- Develops bones and teeth.
- Helps specialized cells. Vitamin A helps epithelial cells develop. These are special cells found in your skin and in the lining of mucous membranes, like those in your throat, digestive system, and of course, your eyes.
- Helps prevent cancer. Experts aren't exactly sure how, but vitamin A, either in its retinol or carotene form, seems to play a crucial role in warding off cancer, especially cancer of the epithelial cells.
- Neutralizes the nasties. Beta-carotene and vitamin A also seem to possess antioxidant properties. Antioxidants hamstring the body's rampaging free radicals, which are unstable molecules that potentially cause everything from cancer to the effects of aging.

Getting the Alpha Vitamin

Here's how to feel A-OK.

Take it easy. Your body excretes some vitamins, like C or B, when you get too much. This isn't necessarily so with vitamin A, which is why doses above 15,000 IU should be taken under medical supervision. In fact, says Musk, getting too much may result in vitamin mortality, rather than vitamin vitality.

"I generally feel that people who take supplements are the people who often need them the least," Musk says. "But with vitamin A, supplements can be even more dangerous.

"I warn people about excess vitamin A intake, which affects the central nervous system and, in extraordinarily large doses, can cause death," Musk says. "Most toxicity occurs through unhealthy and unwise supplementation."

Be careful with beta-carotene. Avoid taking too much beta-carotene, too. Despite its near-mystical appeal, you may look like a walking carrot.

"I've seen this in a few clients of mine," Musk says. "They're drinking too much carrot juice because someone told them to. Too much won't kill them, but it will turn their skin an orange-yellow because all that carotene gets stored in the skin."

Seek a variety of food sources. Not only will you get healthier amounts of vitamin A and beta-carotene that way but also you'll be on the road to an overall healthy diet that will serve you well. Moreover, eating a varied, healthy natural diet—especially one rich in produce—will expose you to more of the carotenes than just beta-carotene.

"This is the reason why I recommend eating a variety of produce. Why limit yourself to just one carotene when you can benefit from many?" Musk says.

Look it up. Although vitamin A deficiency isn't something to worry about in the United States, about half of the more than 80,000 children in Third World nations who go blind each year from a lack of vitamin A eventually die. Make sure to get enough in your diet—but not too much—and be thankful that you can.

Don't let your food get fresh air. Although vitamin A and carotenes are relatively hardy, they do lose potency when exposed to

---

Liver and Let Live

We know that this is asking a lot, but next time you're trekking through the Arctic and are tempted to hunt a polar bear, overcome the urge to fry up its liver after the field dressing.

Since 1596, Arctic explorers have known that dining on polar bear liver, or feeding it to their pack dogs, can be lethal. No one ever knew why until polar bear liver was examined in a laboratory. Then scientists discovered that polar bear liver contains up to 18,000 international units of vitamin A *per gram*. So when a hungry explorer or sled dog eats a modest 500-gram serving, they're consuming a staggering 9,000,000 international units of vitamin A—1,800 times the amount the human body needs in a day, according to the U.S. government, and more than enough to ruin your expedition.

Incidentally, your own liver is where most of your vitamin A is stored. Right now, if you're eating a healthy diet, your liver has enough vitamin A to last you roughly 4 to 12 months. But you can bet that it doesn't have enough to poison a polar bear.

---

the air. Store animal fat products in cold, dark places. And keep fish-liver oils, like cod-liver oil, in dark bottles (also in dark places) to preserve their levels of vitamin A and carotene.

Don't let baby get too much A. Too much vitamin A supplementation taken in the first three months of pregnancy has been linked with birth defects, even when the amount was 4,000 IU, the Recommended Dietary Allowance for women, which is less than half of what you can find in some multivitamins. If your wife or girlfriend is pregnant, make sure that she sticks to the prenatal vitamins that her doctor prescribes to make sure that she's not getting more vitamin A than she needs, warns Musk.

Vitamin B Complex

Think of the B vitamins as the little wooden blocks in the game Jenga, where you attempt to dismantle and then rebuild a tower—piece by piece—without causing a collapse. Without the right piece in the right place, the rest of the tower crumbles or is in danger of crumbling. Only together, in unison, can the separate pieces attain their ultimate goal of working together.

That's a pretty good picture of how the B-complex vitamins work. Yet the B vitamins are so often broken down into their individual pieces that people rarely get to know or appreciate them as a whole. To be sure, those individual pieces are important—vital, even. But, in the case of the B vitamins, you have to see the whole to understand the parts *and* you have to understand the parts to appreciate the whole. But frankly, it's tough to figure out what the parts even are. Some go by letters (B_6, B_{12}), some by names (riboflavin, thiamin). It can all seem so, well, complex.

"Most energy metabolism pathways use one or more of the B vitamins, so you can understand their importance," says Cindy J. Fuller, R.D., Ph.D., assistant professor of food, nutrition, and food service management at the University of North Carolina at Greensboro. "One reason why the B vitamins as a whole are difficult to understand is because they have so many names. The reason is historical."

Here's the history and the mystery of the B vitamins revealed.

Eight Is Enough

Like Dr. Fuller said, the vitamin B family, called the vitamin B complex, can be difficult to understand, in part, because of its many names. So let's start from the beginning.

The vitamin B complex is comprised of eight members. All the B vitamins are water-soluble, meaning that they dissolve in water. Why is that important? Because solubility affects your body's ability to absorb vitamins. Water-soluble vitamins, which include vitamin C and the vitamin B complex, are absorbed directly into the blood. Fat-soluble vitamins aren't.

"In concert, the B vitamins are a fascinating lot in that they're all necessary in fat, carbohydrate, and protein metabolism," says Mara Vitolins, R.D., Dr. P.H., nutrition research coordinator for the Bowman Gray School of Medicine of Wake Forest University in Winston-Salem, North Carolina.

"While you need certain individual B vitamins for specific reasons—niacin, for example, or you run the risk of adverse effects such as fatigue, irritability, or digestive and skin disorders—you also need the B vitamins as a whole," Dr. Vitolins says. In general, the B vitamins are found in green, leafy vegetables and whole grains. "However, B_{12} is unusual because you can only get it from animal products, which is why there are sometimes B_{12} deficiencies in pure vegetarians," Dr. Vitolins says.

"The funny thing is that there are millions of dollars spent every year on vitamin B research, and a lot of the time it comes down to this: You need them all, so Mom was right. Your best approach is to eat a variety of healthy nutritious foods," Dr. Vitolins says.

The role that many of the B vitamins play in the body is what you'd call an official helper-outer. We'll spare you more technical jargon, but suffice it to say that the B vitamins are crucial in providing coenzymes that assist in metabolism. (Coenzymes assist enzymes, protein catalysts that spark vital chemical reactions in the body.) Some B vitamin coenzymes facilitate energy-releasing reactions. Others build new cells to help deliver oxygen and nutrients.

In short, the eight members of the vitamin B complex perform thousands of functions in the body, including the creation of DNA and thus the creation of new cells. Moreover, they act interdependently, meaning, for example, that a lack of riboflavin (one B vitamin) will inhibit the work of vitamin B_6, which needs riboflavin to change into coenzyme form.

"B vitamins, in general, are particularly good for your nervous system, and that's how they'll enhance your functioning," says Richard F. Gerson, Ph.D., a health and fitness consultant in Clearwater, Florida. "But, again, you need the entire B complex. You can't just pick and choose which B vitamins you want to get without doing your body a disservice."

The only problem is that it's hard to tell the B vitamin players without a program. So here it is. On the following pages, we'll detail each of the "Killer Bs" for you.

Folic Acid

• **Where You Get It:** Liver; beans; green, leafy vegetables.

• **What It Does for You:** Helps in DNA synthesis and cell growth, is a major player for red blood cells, and is crucial in creating amino acids.

• **What a Man Needs:** Daily Value of 400 micrograms.

• **Cautions:** Too little can cause anemia and gastrointestinal problems. It's almost impossible to get too much; however, supplementation in amounts greater than 400 micrograms can mask a vitamin B_{12} deficiency.

Next time you're walking through the woods on a crisp autumn afternoon, take a mind-cleansing breath of fresh air and pause under the cobalt blue sky. Then take a gander at the trees and observe nature's palette of colors. The reds, the yellows, the greens, the browns, and all the in-betweens.

Now think of folic acid.

The connection between leaves and the vitamin called folic acid isn't merely a product of our overactive imaginations. It's a real link, one that scientists made decades ago when they discovered folic acid in 1941. A group of researchers in Texas coined the term *folic acid* after finding a mysterious substance in spinach that spurred growth in bacteria. They suspected, correctly, that the substance was widely available in green, leafy plants, so they called it *folic*, from the Latin word *folium*, meaning "foliage or leaf."

Like an autumn leaf, folic acid in its pure form is colorful. It's bright yellow, crystalline, and powdery. It's also unstable, unable to withstand even something as innocuous as light, which destroys it immediately. Yet folic acid is strangely powerful. Without it, *you'd* be destroyed immediately.

Passing the Folic Acid Test

Folic acid—known as folate when it's found naturally in food—is responsible for more than a half-dozen life-sustaining functions in the human body. It's pivotal in creating several types of amino acids, the building blocks of protein and the stuff we're made of. It's also critical in creating heme, the iron-laden substance in hemoglobin. Hemoglobin is the mainstay of red blood cells, which are crucial to every breath we take.

Folic acid plays an important role in cell division and protein synthesis, two functions that you need to live. Without enough folic acid, your cells wouldn't grow or function. One of the first things to falter is red blood cell production. Another thing to go would be your gut. It follows, then, that the first two symptoms of folate deficiency are

The Fickleness of Folic Acid

For such a critical vitamin, folic acid suffers from an identity crisis. It goes by more names than an escaped felon.

Here's a list of folic acid's most commonly used aliases.

- **Folic acid:** The first name given for folate. It's what people generally mean when they talk folates.
- **Folate:** This designates a group of closely related substances. It's the vitamin found naturally in foods and is essential for all animal life.
- **Folacin:** *See* Folate.
- **Pteroylglutamic acid:** The chemical name for folic acid.
- **Wills' factor:** Named after Lucy Wills, an early folic acid researcher in Bombay, India, who, in 1931, discovered that pregnant women with anemia became less anemic after being given yeast.
- **Vitamin M, vitamin B_c, vitamin B_9, vitamin B_{10}, vitamin B_{11}, vitamin U:** Labels given to folate by early researchers.
- **SLR factor, factor R, factor U, *Lactobacillus casei* factor, citrovoram factor, and yeast Norit eluate factor:** Other early names for folate.

generally anemia (where your body produces large but ineffective red blood cells) and stomach problems, including diarrhea, heartburn, and constipation.

Experts are discovering that folic acid might be important to your heart. Researchers in Ottawa, Canada, examined data from more than 5,000 middle-age and older men and women and found that those with the most folic acid were 69 percent less likely to die of heart disease than those with the least folic acid.

"Folate may have some promise in treatment and prevention of heart disease, but all the scientific data are not there yet," says Dr. Fuller. Folate supplementation at the Daily Value level may be appropriate for men with a strong family history of premature heart disease, that is, heart attack before age 50.

Here are some folate-related things that may be of personal interest.

Have a cup. At dinnertime, turn to the right stuff to get most of the folate you need. Your best bets are green, leafy vegetables (especially spinach) and lentils, two of the most folate-packed foods around. A half-cup serving of cooked lentils has nearly all you need for a day, while a cup of cooked spinach packs in almost 50 percent. Other good bean sources are pinto, navy, lima, and kidney beans.

Keep it fresh. Cooking kills between 50 and 95 percent of your food's folate. While you shouldn't lose a tooth filling crunching on uncooked kidney beans, avoid cooking folate-rich food whenever possible, or cook it as little as possible. Lightly steam, instead of boiling, your broccoli, or consider a fresh spinach salad instead of boiling it as a side dish.

Don't wait for folate. Folic acid is not a fine wine. It doesn't improve with age. Raw vegetables stored at room temperature for two to three days may lose 50 to 70 percent of their folate.

Don't let your folate go up in smoke. Smoking retards your body's ability to use folic acid, especially in a localized way. It has been shown that smokers' lungs show a localized deficiency compared to the lungs of nonsmokers. Reason Number 6,770 to quit. Certain drugs such as aspirin and antacids also can inhibit folic acid. Most healthy adults eating a good diet shouldn't worry about taking an occasional aspirin or antacid, but chronic users, such as arthritis and ulcer sufferers, should question their doctors.

Vitamin B$_6$

• **Where You Get It:** Rice bran, wheat bran, sunflower seeds, avocados, bananas, lean meat, fish, corn, brown rice, whole grains.

• **What It Does for You:** Helps metabolize protein, carbohydrates, and fats. Involved with hemoglobin formation, the absorption of amino acids, and the central nervous system.

• **What a Man Needs:** Daily Value of 2 milligrams.

• **Cautions:** Too little can cause irritability, depression, muscle weakness, and greasy scaliness of the skin around the eyes, nose, and mouth. Too much is nearly impossible, but megadoses of 50 milligrams to 2 grams daily can result in an unstable gait, numb feet, sleepiness, and physiologic dependence when taken over the long haul.

As you're probably learning is the case with many vitamins, vitamin B$_6$ isn't just one substance. It's actually three chemically similar substances—pyridoxine, pyridoxal, and pyridoxamine—collectively called B$_6$, by virtue of international agreement. Its need was first demonstrated in laboratory rats, and it has since been found necessary to sustain life in pigs, chicks, dogs, and other animal species, including microorganisms and, of course, humans.

The key breakthrough in discovering B$_6$ came in 1926, when two scientists tried to reproduce pellagra in rats. (Pellagra, from *pelle*, meaning "skin," and *agra*, meaning "rough," is a vitamin B deficiency marked by scaly, flaky

dark skin; dementia; and diarrhea.) They succeeded, and eight years later a Hungarian scientist produced a cure from yeast extract. The substance extracted was not one of the recognized B vitamins—niacin, riboflavin, or thiamin—so he named it vitamin B$_6$. By 1940, five independent laboratories, working alone, isolated vitamin B$_6$ in crystalline form; it was also called pyridoxine, after its chemical makeup. Two years later, further research revealed two similar substances, which were named pyridoxal and pyridoxamine.

Today, we know that all three white crystalline substances are rightfully called vitamin B$_6$. We also know that these compounds are easily absorbed in the upper part of the small intestine and are present in almost all body tissue, with a high concentration in the liver. They're secreted into milk during lactation and excreted primarily through urine. Vitamin B$_6$ is easily dissolved in water, quite resistant to heat and acid, but easily destroyed by oxidation, exposure to alkalis, and ultraviolet light.

Of the three forms, pyridoxine is the most resistant to food processing and storage conditions and is probably the form that you're getting most in your food.

As for what vitamin B$_6$ does, the question is more like what it doesn't do. B$_6$ is involved in a large number of physiologic activities, many of which are crucial to survival. Vitamin B$_6$ plays a large role in protein metabolism, helps form hemoglobin, and aids in absorbing amino acids from the intestine. It also plays a part in metabolizing fat and carbohydrates. Moreover, scientists have linked vitamin B$_6$, or the lack thereof, to several clinical maladies, including the following:

• Central nervous system breakdowns. Vitamin B$_6$ helps with energy transformation in the brain and nerve tissue. When it's lacking, the result can be convulsive seizures.
• Autism. Although more research is needed, a number of experiments show

promise that megadoses of vitamin B_6 under a doctor's supervision may ameliorate autism, a severe disturbance of mental and emotional development in young children.

- Kidney stones. Lack of vitamin B_6 has been linked to an increased formation of kidney stones.

Here's more on how to make the most of vitamin B_6.

Watch for losses. Wheat loses more than 75 percent of its vitamin B_6 when it's milled into white flour. Beef loses 25 to 50 percent of its B_6 stores when it's cooked (more through oven braising than oven roasting.) And cooking vegetables and fruits at home results in losses of 50 percent or more. Keep this in mind next time you make a B_6-conscious eating decision—the less processed your food, the better it will be B-wise.

De-emphasize diabetes damage. If you have diabetes—and some 7.2 million American men do—then ask your doctor about vitamin B_6 supplements. "People with diabetes experience less of the numbness and tingling of diabetes-related nerve damage if they get supplements of B vitamins, most notably B_6," says John Marion Ellis, M.D., a retired physician in Mount Pleasant, Texas, who spent most of his professional life researching vitamin B_6.

See the light at the end of the carpal tunnel. If your job has you pounding a keyboard for 8 hours a day—or doing any other repetitive task for hours on end, like working on an assembly line—then you have a vested interest in knowing more about vitamin B_6 because it may be helpful in preventing carpal tunnel syndrome.

"You couldn't say enough about carpal tunnel and vitamin B_6—the evidence is that positive," says Dr. Ellis. He contends that the swelling and inelasticity of the sheath surrounding nerves in the wrist may be caused by a lack of vitamin B_6.

Get to the meat of the matter. About 41 percent of all available vitamin B_6 comes from meat, poultry, and fish. That's not to say that you should overdo it on the meat or that there isn't a world of good from a diet rich in vegetables. But it's something to keep in mind when someone castigates you for enjoying your once-a-month rib eye.

Vitamin B_{12}

- ***Where You Get It:*** Liver and organ meats, muscle meats, shellfish, eggs, cheese, fish.

- ***What It Does for You:*** Aids in red blood cell formation and in the prevention of pernicious anemia (impaired absorption of vitamin B_{12} in the intestine), maintains nerve tissue, and helps metabolize carbohydrates, fats, and proteins.

- ***What a Man Needs:*** Daily Value of 6 micrograms.

- ***Cautions:*** Too little, sometimes seen in strict vegetarians, can cause sore tongue, weakness, weight loss, back pain, and apathy. There are no known toxic effects from too much—leftovers are excreted through urine.

Like vitamin B_6, vitamin B_{12} isn't just one substance. It's actually several compounds, all of which contain cobalt, giving them the generic name of cobalamins. When not otherwise indicated, the substance assumed to be in question when talk turns to B_{12} is cyanocobalamin, the most active compound. The other compounds are hydroxocobalamin, nitritocobalamin, and thiocyanate cobalamin.

As you'd probably guess from its tongue-twisting names, B_{12} has the distinct honor of having the largest and most complex chemical structure of any vitamin known to man. Just looking at a diagram of its chemical components is dizzying, so you can imagine the enigma that it presented to early researchers.

The first B_{12} research was the result of work by Thomas Addison, a London physician, who first described an illness that was later determined to come from a lack of B_{12}. Dr. Addison described in 1849 a type of anemia that progressed slowly and killed its victims in two to five years. It was so insidious that it was described as pernicious anemia and later became known as Addisonian pernicious anemia in his honor. It took more than 70 years for something to be done about pernicious anemia, starting in 1925 with research by George Hoyt Whipple, M.D., former dean of the University of Rochester School of Medicine and Dentistry in New York. Dr. Whipple showed that liver was beneficial in treating anemia in dogs. A year later, two researchers from Harvard Medical School elaborated on Dr. Whipple's findings, determining that ¼ to ½ pound of raw liver a day overcame pernicious anemia. For their discoveries, they and Dr. Whipple were awarded the Nobel prize in 1934.

It wasn't until 1948, however, that researchers isolated a red, crystalline substance that they called vitamin B_{12} from a liver. Later that same year, researchers at Columbia University in New York City found that B_{12} abated pernicious anemia, and seven years later, a second Nobel prize was awarded for B_{12} research, this time going to Dorothy Hodgkin and co-workers at Oxford University in England, for deciphering the complex chemical structure of B_{12}.

Today, we know many more fascinating things about B_{12}. Unlike any other vitamin, it cannot be synthesized by plants, which is why it's found almost exclusively in meat and meat products. It is the only vitamin that requires specific juices from your gastrointestinal tract to be absorbed. And B_{12} absorption takes a remarkably long time—about 3 hours, compared to just seconds for other water-soluble vitamins.

Moreover, vitamin B_{12} is remarkably potent and durable. In the cooking process, only 30 percent of a food's B_{12} content may be lost. Its synthetic form has a potency level some 11,000 times that found in the standard liver concentrate once used to treat pernicious anemia. Deficiencies of vitamin B_{12} have been linked to two major areas of health concerns. They are:

• Central nervous system problems. A raft of problems have been linked to vitamin B_{12} deficiencies, including memory loss, confusion, delusion, fatigue, loss of balance, decreased reflexes, numbness and tingling in the hands, and ringing in the ears. It has also been linked to multiple sclerosis–like symptoms and dementia. "In a severe deficiency, there is actually a degeneration of the myelin sheath. The stuff begins to literally erode," says John Pinto, Ph.D., director of the nutrition research laboratory at Memorial Sloan-Kettering Cancer Center and associate professor of biochemistry at Cornell University Medical College, both in New York City. (Myelin is a fatty sheath of tissue that insulates nerve fibers, keeping electrical pulses humming through your body.)

• Dangerous chemical imbalance. Research shows that a lack of B_{12} raises the levels of a substance called homocysteine. Homocysteine, in high doses, is toxic to the brain, raising questions about its potential role in Alzheimer's disease; it has also been suggested as a primary cause of heart disease.

Here's how not to be a B_{12} bomber when it comes to getting the nutrition you need.

Be a dairy king. Pure vegans—people who eat only plant foods—may be seriously deficient in vitamin B_{12}. But if you stopped eating foods that contain B_{12} today, it might take up to 20 years to show signs of deficiency. That's because your body will continue to recycle its B_{12} for as long as it can, reabsorbing it over and over. And even when that stops happening, it will take some 3 years to deplete your body's extreme emergency conservation supplies.

If you opt for a vegetarian lifestyle, consider being a lacto-ovo vegetarian, meaning that you permit yourself eggs and milk. (Just 1 cup of milk, one egg, or 3½ ounces of cheese a day is all you need to protect against B_{12} deficiency.) Or, says Dr. Vitolins, include meat replacement foods in your diet, like vegetarian burgers, which are textured vegetable-protein products fortified with nutrients often found in real meat.

Don't hit the bottle. As if you'd really need a reason not to drink excessively, here's one vitamin-wise: Excess alcohol, especially when coupled with an unhealthy diet, can rob your body of B vitamins, especially B_{12}, according to international nutrition consultant Maye Musk. "The men who have come to see me have not been alcoholics. They may have been heavy drinkers, but they wanted to follow a healthy lifestyle," Musk adds. "They can by making better food choices and drinking less."

Don't let your B_{12} dry up. Milk is a good source of B_{12}, as we mentioned before. But stick to regular, low-fat milk. Pasteurization results in a loss of only 10 percent of B_{12}, whereas evaporated milk loses up to 90 percent of its B_{12}.

Add B_{12} as you age. Because the inner workings of your gut change as you grow older, there's serious concern that there might be a grand-scale B_{12} deficiency among the elderly. Even when they do eat meat and drink milk, up to one-third of all people over 60 can't extract the B_{12} they need from their food because their stomachs no longer produce enough gastric acid. (Remember that B_{12} requires specific gastric juices to be absorbed.) If you're over age 60, or have a loved one who is, ask your doctor about the feasibility of getting a B_{12} shot or using supplementation to curb these effects.

Get it in food. It's easy to put away a health food store–size helping of B_{12} and not get sick—in simply eating your meals. Vitamin B_{12} has no known toxic effects, and because it's easy to get adequate amounts of B_{12} from food

alone, there's probably no need to take a B_{12} supplement unless you're told to do so by your doctor.

"B vitamins are widespread in healthy diets. If a B vitamin is lacking, it's probably because your diet is poor," says Musk.

Thiamin (Vitamin B_1)

• **Where You Get It:** Enriched cornflakes, sunflower seeds, peanuts, wheat bran, enriched rice, enriched white bread, beef liver, egg yolk, lima beans, refried beans.

• **What It Does for You:** Necessary component in energy metabolism, nerve maintenance and functioning, and muscle maintenance and functioning. Maintains healthy appetite and healthy mental attitude.

• **What a Man Needs:** Daily Value of 1.5 milligrams.

• **Cautions:** Too little can lead to fatigue, apathy, loss of appetite, depression, and numbness in legs. Extreme deficiency can lead to beriberi, a serious inflammation of the nerves. No known toxic effects.

When it comes to turning the starches and sugars in your breakfast bowl into energy that your body can use, this vitamin is number one. Or, to be precise, number B_1. But you can just call it thiamin.

Discovered during the long years of research that led to a cure for beriberi, this vitamin was first dubbed water-soluble B by researcher Elmer V. McCollum of the

University of Wisconsin in 1916. Ten years later, two researchers in Holland isolated the exact chemical, which, in 1936, was chemically identified and synthesized by American Robert R. Williams, who named it *thiamine,* because it contained sulfur, from *thio,* meaning "sulfur-containing," and *amine,* the name for organic compounds derived from ammonia. (The final "e" was later dropped.)

Since then, we've learned a lot more about this beriberi-important vitamin, including the following:

- Thiamin is a crystalline white powder, with a faint yeastlike odor and a salty, nutty taste.

- Thiamin is the least stored vitamin in the body. Your liver, kidneys, heart, brain, and muscles hold the most, but there's still only about 30 milligrams total in the entire body. Moreover, your thiamin reserve can be depleted in just one to two weeks without continual reinforcement.

- Thiamin provides one of the most miraculous cures known to modern medicine. A patient ridden with wet beriberi can lie in bed, apparently dying, breathless, and virtually drowning from edema, an internal accumulation of body fluids. But within 2 hours after being given a thiamin injection, that patient can be back on his feet, almost fully recovered.

- Thiamin is necessary for muscle tone and nerve function. It's also responsible for energy production, for without thiamin, there could be no metabolic energy. Likewise, it plays a critical role in maintaining a healthy mental attitude.

"If you dramatically reduce thiamin intake, you reduce the ability of the brain to use glucose and to make neurotransmitters. And if you reduce that, you have impaired mental function," says Gary E. Gibson, Ph.D., professor of neuroscience at Cornell University Medical College's Burke Medical Research In-stitute in White Plains, New York.

Here are details on getting more thiamin.

Eat extra well if you're active. Active bodies need more energy (and thus more food) than sedentary ones. Make doubly sure that your diet is rich in an array of healthy foods and is especially heavy on the grains, fruits, and vegetables. The healthier food you'll be eating should ensure that you're getting enough thiamin to keep you active.

Pour a bowl of thiamin in the morning. Breakfast cereal is commonly fortified with thiamin and other nutrients, making it a good way to start the day. Ditto for enriched and whole-grain breads, which make a nice complement to healthy cereal. Since the U.S. government began the enrichment plan for flour and bread in 1941, more than 40 percent of every person's daily requirement of thiamin is supplied by these foods.

Start your own microbrew. Home-brewed beer and wine may contain significant amounts of thiamin. That's because the yeast used in fermenting is thiamin-rich, and likely to remain residually, making your brew a potentially potent elixir of thiamin. (Some African and Latin American communities derive most of their thiamin from native beer.) Just don't use this as a cheap excuse to hoist another round at the local watering hole next Friday—commercial beers are void of thiamin-rich yeast.

Convert now. Converted rice, that is, rice that's soaked and parboiled, is a better source of thiamin than rice that was milled from its raw state. Parboiling causes thiamin and other water-soluble nutrients to move from the outer layers to the inner layers of the rice kernel, so fewer of them are removed in the milling process.

Don't add soda to preserve the green. There's an old wives' tale that adding baking soda to the water in which you're boiling green vegetables will preserve their color. Maybe so, but it kills their thiamin. Baking soda is an alkali, and alkalies easily de-stroy thiamin.

Riboflavin (Vitamin B₂)

• **Where You Get It:** Organ meats, enriched cornflakes, almonds, cheese, eggs, lean meats (beef, pork, lamb), enriched white bread, milk.

• **What It Does for You:** Helps the body use oxygen; assists in metabolizing amino acids, fatty acids, and carbohydrates; helps activate vitamin B₆; helps create niacin (vitamin B₃); and aids the adrenal gland.

• **What a Man Needs:** Daily Value of 1.7 milligrams.

• **Cautions:** Too little isn't much danger but can contribute to other B vitamin deficiencies. Some deficiency symptoms include sore, swollen, chapped lips; painful tongue; oily, scaly skin; and redness and congestion of the cornea. No known toxicity.

Riboflavin's roots lie in milk scum. Maybe that sounds pretty gross, but it's not far from the truth. Pure riboflavin was first isolated in 1933 by a German scientist from milk as part of an ongoing process to identify a yellow-green fluorescent substance in milk whey that had been identified as early as the late 1800s. The substance had previously been identified as some type of pigment—a pigment subsequently found in a variety of other sources, including liver, heart, and egg whites. Called flavin, the pigment remained an enigma to researchers, who couldn't find a biological reason for its existence.

It wasn't until the mid-1930s, thanks largely to German and Swiss researchers, that scientists learned more about this mysterious pigment, which was later named riboflavin because it has ribitol as part of its flavin chemical structure.

Not much has changed since then. Unlike research on the other B vitamins during that era—and research on the antioxidant darlings of today (A, C, and E)—riboflavin research has remained fairly low-key. "It's not fashionable per se, but you're going to be hearing more about it," says Jack M. Cooperman, Ph.D., clinical professor of community and preventive medicine at New York Medical College in Valhalla. "The key concept to remember here is that riboflavin is one of the essential B vitamins necessary for antioxidant activity inside the body."

We know today that riboflavin is absorbed in the small intestine and that the body has a limited capacity for storing it. What little is stored is stored in the liver and kidneys. Whatever else the body needs must be taken in on a daily basis through diet. Leftovers are primarily excreted through the urine. In pure form, riboflavin looks like fine orange-yellow crystals, bitter-tasting and virtually odorless. In water-based solutions, they impart a strange green-yellow glow. Riboflavin is easily destroyed by light, which is partly why milk isn't stored in clear, glass bottles anymore.

In the body, riboflavin's main role is in energy release, which it accomplishes along with a group of enzymes called flavoproteins. Riboflavin is also thought to be a component in the retinal pigment in the eye, involved in the function of the adrenal gland and in the production of corticosteroids in the adrenal cortex.

Here's how to maximize your riboflavin for ultimate vitamin vitality.

Don't make special attempts. Unless you're reading this from a mud hut in a Third World country, you won't need to make a special attempt to get more riboflavin in your diet. Most people easily meet their recommended amounts. The average person gets one-half of his riboflavin from milk and milk products, one-fourth from meats, and the rest from green vegetables, whole-grain or enriched bread, and cereal products.

Choose cartons when you can.
When you buy your milk, choose cardboard cartons. They won't let riboflavin-robbing light in. Opaque plastic jugs work well, too, but avoid glass bottles and other clear containers. Two hours of light can destroy 50 percent or more of milk's riboflavin.

Raise a glass to riboflavin. Reason Number 782,563 to drink a glass of beer once in awhile: Riboflavin is the only vitamin found in significant amounts in beer. One liter will almost take care of your average daily requirement.

Niacin

• *Where You Get It:* Liver, lean meats, poultry, fish, rabbit, enriched cornflakes, nuts, peanut butter, milk, cheese, eggs, sunflower seeds.

• *What It Does for You:* Serves as important coenzyme necessary for cell respiration. Helps release energy from carbohydrates, fats, and proteins. Aids growth, reduces cholesterol, and may protect against heart attack.

• *What a Man Needs:* Daily Value of 20 milligrams.

• *Cautions:* Too little can cause pellagra. Too much is usually not seen, except when given medicinally. Large doses, over 100 milligrams, should only be taken under medical supervision because they can cause flushing of the skin, itching, liver damage, elevated blood glucose, and peptic ulcers.

Niacin's discovery came almost single-handedly from mankind's fight against pellagra, a disease that results in diarrhea, dementia, and a darkening flaking away of the skin. Initially uncommon in Europe, pellagra was first described by Spanish physician Gaspar Casal in 1730, soon after corn was introduced to the European diet. By the nineteenth century, pellagra was widespread in Europe, Africa, and the Americas, particularly in the impoverished, post–Civil War South, where corn was the only sustenance widely available. So widespread and insidious was pellagra that doctors thought it was caused by an infectious agent or a toxic substance found in spoiled corn.

In a strange twist, the cure for pellagra—niacin—was discovered in 1867 by a German chemist, who extracted nicotinic acid (a natural form of niacin) from nicotine in tobacco. However, it would be another 70 years before the connection between niacin and pellagra would be made. By the early 1900s, pellagra had reached epidemic proportions in the southern United States, killing 10,000 people in 1915 and accounting for some 200,000 cases between 1917 and 1918.

In 1914, the U.S. Public Health Service dispatched a team of physicians and researchers to find a cure. By 1925, Joseph Goldberger, M.D., the initiative's leader, found that pellagra resulted from a dietary deficiency, not an infectious agent, and that certain foods—notably yeast, lean meats, and milk—helped prevent it. By 1937, thanks to the initial pioneering, researchers at the University of Wisconsin discovered that two substances, collectively called niacin, were essential when it came to preventing pellagra.

Today, nutritionists know that niacin is actually a collective name for two essential substances, nicotinic acid and nicotinamide, both natural forms of niacin. Since this discovery, pellagra is rare in the United States. It's also rare in Latin American countries and Mexico, despite the prevalence of corn in their diets. This rarity stems from the ancient Mexican tradition of soaking corn flour in lime water to make it easier to knead. This process releases the corn's niacin, which would otherwise be chemically bound and inaccessible to the body. Africa is the only continent where pellagra remains a public health concern.

Biologically, little niacin is stored in the body. Your body uses what it needs and excretes the rest in urine. What is used goes toward energy metabolism. It also seems helpful in lowering cholesterol, though its boon here is a double-edged sword.

"In the right hands, it's very useful medication. It lowers harmful cholesterol and raises good cholesterol better than any drug we have," says James McKenney, Pharm.D., professor of pharmacy at Virginia Commonwealth University Medical College of Virginia School of Pharmacy in Richmond. "But taken indiscriminately by an uninformed person without a professional monitoring his condition, it can be dangerous."

According to Robert C. Atkins, M.D., founder and director of the Atkins Center for Complementary Medicine in New York City who publishes *Dr. Atkins' Health Revelations* newsletter, a daily dose of 1,500 to 3,000 milligrams can reduce low-density lipoprotein (LDL) cholesterol (the "bad" kind) by 10 to 25 percent, while raising high-density lipoprotein (HDL) cholesterol (the "good" kind) by 15 to 35 percent. However, supplementing at these high doses should only be attempted under strict medical supervision.

Large doses of nicotinic acid have a drug-like effect on the nervous system and on the blood. They can dilate blood vessels so much that you feel a tingling sensation, sometimes painful, known as a niacin flush. (The nicotinamide form of niacin doesn't have this effect.) High doses of niacin may also damage the liver and possibly produce diabetes.

Here's what you need to know about niacin.

Take top natural sources. Aim to get most of your required niacin from natural sources. Prized picks include beef liver, tuna (in water), mushrooms, chicken breast, salmon, and asparagus.

Go easy on the water. Because niacin, like all B vitamins, is water-soluble, some 15 to 25 percent of it can disappear quickly if you're cooking with water. That said, it's the most stable of the B vitamins and will otherwise remain resistant to just about every type of food preparation you're bound to do on a given day.

Serve up cereal. Cereal and cereal products are fair sources of niacin because the government in the 1940s mandated that these products be fortified with niacin. Ditto for enriched white flour. (Incidentally, thiamin and riboflavin are added, too.)

Pour a strong cup of niacin. Coffee is a good source of niacin—a cup of dark-roast alone provides some 3 milligrams. In some areas of the world, where diets are low in niacin, a large consumption of coffee is thought to prevent widespread cases of pellagra.

Biotin

• **Where You Get It:** Cheese, beef liver, cauliflower, eggs, mushrooms, chicken breast, salmon, spinach.

• **What It Does for You:** Metabolizes fats, proteins, and carbohydrates; helps in the transfer of carbon dioxide; and assists in various metabolic chemical conversions.

• **What a Man Needs:** Daily Value of 300 micrograms.

• **Cautions:** Too little can lead to dry, scaly skin; loss of appetite; vomiting; nausea; mental depression; tongue inflammation; and high cholesterol. No known toxic effects.

Biotin plays an important role in metabolism by acting as a coenzyme that helps transport carbon dioxide from compound to compound. (Coenzymes assist enzymes in making metabolic reactions come to fruition.) It also helps convert various substances that are chemically important in processes like protein synthesis, the formation of long-chain fatty acids, and in the Krebs cycle, which is the process that releases energy from foods.

The average U.S. biotin intake is estimated to be 100 to 300 micrograms a day, and you're probably getting all you need by eating a healthy, well-rounded diet.

"The people who need to worry about biotin most are bodybuilders who eat raw eggs," says Musk. The reason is because raw eggs contain a biotin-binding substance called avidin. That can keep the body from absorbing the biotin it needs. "It's rare and I've never come across it, but it happens," Musk says. There are no known toxic levels of biotin.

Pantothenic Acid

• **Where You Get It:** Liver, wheat bran, rice bran, nuts, mushrooms, soybean flour, salmon, blue cheese, eggs, brown rice, lobster.

• **What It Does for You:** Helps create energy by breaking down fats, proteins, and carbohydrates; helps form a substance that is important in transmitting nerve impulses; and helps synthesize cholesterol and steroid hormones formed in the adrenal gland.

• **What a Man Needs:** Daily Value of 10 milligrams.

• **Cautions:** Too little leads to irritability, loss of appetite, abdominal pains, nausea, headache, mental depression, fatigue and weakness, muscle cramps, tingling in hands and feet, insomnia, respiratory

infections, and a staggering gait. Doses of 10,000 to 20,000 milligrams per day are not toxic but can cause occasional diarrhea and water retention.

Pantothenic acid is involved in more than 100 different steps in the creation of lipids, neurotransmitters, steroid hormones, and hemoglobin. It's also a factor in growth and is essential for human life. Moreover, pantothenic acid is common, found in many foods. (Its name comes from the Greek word *pantothen*, meaning "everywhere.")

Pantothentic acid functions in the body as part of two enzymes, indirectly aiding in the building and breakdown of fatty acids; the creation of antibodies; the metabolism of fats, proteins, and carbohydrates; and energy metabolism. It's also influential on the endocrine glands and the hormones they produce.

Though found in many foods, pantothenic acid has one major drawback: It's easily destroyed in massive amounts by food processing. A study done at Dartmouth Medical School in Hanover, New Hampshire, found that 58 percent is lost from milling wheat into all-purpose flour; up to 79 percent is lost by canning vegetables; and just over 26 percent is lost by canning meat and poultry. Canning seafood destroys almost 20 percent of the pantothenic acid.

Here are a couple of other things to keep in mind about pantothenic acid.

Stick to cereal grains. Pantothenic acid is reasonably stable in natural foods during storage. Some cereal grains may be kept for up to a year without appreciable loss.

Gut it out. Sticking to a healthy diet and lifestyle ensures that your intestinal flora—the bacteria naturally occurring in your gut—stay healthy. That's important when it comes to pantothenic acid because it is synthesized by intestinal bacteria. However, scientists aren't sure how much pantothenic acid is produced by the body or how much is used, a strong argument in favor of doing all you can to keep those bacteria buggers—and the rest of you—healthy.

Vitamin C

• ***Where You Get It:*** Green, leafy vegetables (broccoli, brussels sprouts); red cabbage; citrus fruits (oranges, grapefruits, lemons); guavas; parsley; mustard greens.

• ***What It Does for You:*** Helps form and maintain collagen. Is an excellent wound healer. Metabolizes amino acids, fats, and lipids. Helps iron absorption. Promotes strong teeth, bones, and capillary walls. Possibly boosts immunity and prevents colds, infections, and cancer.

• ***What a Man Needs:*** Daily Value of 60 milligrams, 100 milligrams a day if he smokes.

• ***Cautions:*** Too little causes scurvy, which may lead to massive internal bleeding and heart failure. Too much is hard to do, but side effects, reported at levels more than 33 times the Daily Value, include cramps, nausea, diarrhea, destruction of red blood cells, and kidney and bladder stone formation.

In today's world, James Lind's brand of science wouldn't get past the gate guard at a major university. Yet Lind, a British naval surgeon who lived in the mid-1700s, is responsible for discovering the most compelling thing we know about vitamin C today: Without it, you die a slow, painful, bloody death.

Lind's early experiments with vitamin C hardly met today's scientific criteria. It wasn't what you'd call a randomized, controlled, double-blind clinical trial, the gold standard of modern testing. "In other words, from the scientific communities' standpoint, there was no sig-

nificant compelling evidence," says Dr. Michael Janson of the American Preventive Medicine Association and the Center for Preventive Medicine.

Lind tested six pairs of sailors ravaged by scurvy, a vitamin C deficiency that literally destroys the body from the inside out. (Of course, no one knew that at the time.) He treated each pair with doses of either cider, vinegar, sulfuric acid, seawater, oranges and lemons, or a spice mixture. Sailors treated with the citrus fruits recovered within a week. The rest, presumably, wound up resting with Davy Jones on the ocean floor. Despite their promise, Lind's findings weren't published for 6 years. More astonishing, they weren't put to use for another 50 years.

The Old Man and the C

Vitamin C today is perhaps the most widely studied vitamin. It gets its scientific name, ascorbic acid, from "anti-scurvy acid." Of all substances in Nutritionland, it's the reigning media darling, thought to reduce the risk of heart disease, reverse aging, bolster the immune system, strengthen bones, fight cancer, treat asthma, and even cure the common cold, depending, of course, on what you read or to whom you talk.

Yet for something that has attracted so much attention and so many devotees, vitamin C could have used a better public relations man because it—or, rather, its deficiency—has been known since 1550 B.C. Scurvy symptoms were described then on medical papyrus rolls discovered in Thebes by George Moritz Ebers, a nineteenth-century "Indiana Jones" and novelist. Descriptions of vitamin C deficiency also make appearances in the Bible's Old Testament; the writings of Hippocrates, the father of modern medicine; a chronicle of the Crusades; and the logbooks of Vasco da Gama, the Portuguese sailor who established the first European trading colony. Da Gama reported losing to scurvy 100 of his 160-man crew on one trip alone.

In time—thanks, in part, to Lind—sailors everywhere began to recognize the importance of vegetables and citrus juice in preventing scurvy. In 1795, the British Navy mandated that all their sailors get a 1-ounce serving of lime juice daily, earning them the nickname "limeys." This practice grew and more experiments were conducted, though it wasn't until 1932 that vitamin C itself was discovered. Charles Glen King at the University of Pittsburgh then answered the age-old question of what exactly cured scurvy by isolating a crystalline substance from lemon juice.

Thanks to all the down-and-dirty research through the centuries—and lots of lost teeth and bleeding gums—a vitamin, and thus a nutritional sensation, was born.

How It Works

As it turns out, the ravages of vitamin C deficiency aren't a disease at all. Scientists have learned since that humans and certain other animals need vitamin C because of a genetic shortcoming.

Man, monkeys, guinea pigs, fruit-eating bats, and certain birds lack a gene responsible for producing oxidase, an enzyme that otherwise would permit us to live fulfilling lives without ingesting vitamin C in our food. This is precisely why your son's garter snake doesn't need fruits and vegetables to say "fangs" for dinner.

Inside your body, vitamin C does a lot of good. It's crucial in creating and maintaining collagen, a fibrous protein that binds cells together much like mortar binds bricks. Consequently, vitamin C is an incomparable ally in healing wounds and burns and in strengthening the walls of capillaries and blood vessels. Vitamin C also helps metabolize the amino

Meet Linus of the C-nuts

Early vitamin C pioneer Linus Pauling, Ph.D., is one of history's rare overachievers. He was a respected chemist and a winner of two—count 'em, two—unshared Nobel prizes: one in 1954 for chemistry, the other in 1962 for peace. He is also the father of the vitamin C movement.

Dr. Pauling wrote his seminal best-seller *Vitamin C and the Common Cold* in 1970 and, with it, started the craze for vitamin C. He further fired the C frenzy by finding that vitamin C–treated terminal patients lived four times longer than patients not receiving the vitamin. Dr. Pauling's study involved 1,100 cancer victims, 100 of whom were given 10,000 milligrams of vitamin C a day. Even one year after he published his results, Dr. Pauling said, "Thirteen of these 'hopeless' patients are still alive, some as long as five years after having been pronounced untreatable, and most of them are in such good apparent health as to suggest that they now have normal life expectancy."

Dr. Pauling himself took 12,000 milligrams of vitamin C in his orange juice every morning, enjoying enviable health up to the age of 93, when he died just one year after weathering a bout of prostate cancer, something he says that he postponed for decades by taking vitamin C. After all, Dr. Pauling never said that vitamin C makes you immortal—just healthier.

acids tyrosine and tryptophan, increase the absorption of iron, promote sound teeth and bones, and quite possibly, stave off infection, common colds, and even cancer.

How does vitamin C do all these wondrous things? Scientists aren't exactly certain, and research continues. But they're reasonably sure that part of it is because of vitamin C's well-established antioxidant properties. Antioxidants are substances that neutralize free radicals—Tasmanian devil–like, rogue molecules thought to cause everything from the ravages of aging to cancer.

"Not that all free radicals are bad. White blood cells, for example, use them like bullets in fighting foreign invaders," Dr. Janson says.

"Free radicals are like sparks in your fireplace. They're okay as long as they stay where they're supposed to stay. Once they get on the living room rug, there's trouble," he adds.

Vitamin C and other antioxidants tame beastly free radicals by offering up one of their electrons to neutralize the buggers. That way, free radicals don't prey on electrons from the body's healthy molecules.

"If the free radicals were like the sparks from the fireplace, vitamin C and other antioxidants would be like the asbestos gloves you'd wear to handle them," Dr. Janson says.

Health and fitness consultant Dr. Richard F. Gerson has heard the "Pac-Man" analogy applied to vitamin C and other antioxidants. Under this theory, vitamin C and other antioxidants are likened to the star of the computer game of the same name, where a voracious little creature gobbles everything in sight. Antioxidants, as the theory goes, similarly scoff up free radicals as fast as can be. Dr. Gerson prefers a more constructive, empowering perspective.

"I'd rather look at vitamin C and the others as builders. By taking them and keeping a good healthy diet, you're building a defense against things that could go wrong," Dr. Gerson says.

Regardless of how you view antioxidants, it begs the question: Can you get too much of a good thing?

With vitamin C, probably not. Dr. Gerson, for example, takes 1,000 to 5,000 milligrams a day. And Dr. Janson? As much as 13,000 to 14,000 milligrams a day, although he doesn't

> ## More C, Please
>
> The U.S. government may finally vindicate researchers and scientists who have been carrying the torch for vitamin C.
>
> The current Daily Value of 60 milligrams a day is too low, according to a study performed by the National Institutes of Health (NIH) in Bethesda, Maryland. Subjects were given different doses of vitamin C over time, ranging from 30 milligrams to 2,500 milligrams a day.
>
> When researchers observed their immune system cells and blood, they found that they appeared to be optimally saturated with vitamin C at a daily dose of 200 milligrams. Perhaps more interesting, they found that at

routinely recommend that dose to others.

And why not? "Because based on what I know about vitamins and what I know about myself, it's a reasonable experiment to make," Dr. Janson says.

But doses akin to what early vitamin C pioneer and double Nobel prize winner Dr. Linus Pauling took or the doses Dr. Janson takes aren't recommended by everybody. "While there certainly is a wide range of supplement levels out there, I don't recommend that my clients go above 500 milligrams," says international nutrition consultant Maye Musk.

You need only 10 milligrams to avoid scurvy. If you take 100 times that amount, you might run into adverse reactions such as diarrhea. Taking 2,000 milligrams or more can lead to cramps, nausea, destruction of red blood cells, and even the creation of kidney and bladder stones in people who are prone to them.

Going to the Right Source

Getting the vitamin C that you need is easy. "And if nothing else, taking a reasonable

doses of 400 milligrams and more a day, the subjects retained no more vitamin C in their cells than they did at 200 milligrams.

"It's almost as if we're programmed to have a certain amount of vitamin C and no more," says Mark Levine, M.D., the study's lead researcher. "We don't recommend daily doses higher than 500 milligrams a day."

The NIH study and its recommendations carry a lot of weight. As for exactly when the government will increase its vitamin C recommendations, stay tuned.

amount of vitamins and minerals might have a placebo effect," Dr. Gerson says, meaning that something good might happen just because you *think* something good might happen.

Here's how C-ing is believing.

Seek food sources first. Getting your vitamin C from food sources is a good idea if only because you'll be on the path to an all-around healthy diet. The best vitamin C sources—green, leafy vegetables and citrus fruits—are healthy for many reasons, including being low in fat and high in fiber.

"The only surefire reality in the world, besides death and taxes, is the fact that baby boomers will never grow old gracefully," Dr. Gerson says. "By sticking to a healthy diet, you'll be getting vitamin C and doing many other good things for your body that will keep you healthy and maybe even looking and feeling younger than you really are."

A single serving of broccoli, green peppers, cauliflower, cantaloupe, or strawberries provides more than 50 milligrams of vitamin C for fewer than 60 calories. Other excellent food sources include papaya (more than 180 milligrams!), orange juice, and grapefruit juice.

C is for "care." Handle vitamin C with care, since it's water-soluble and easily destroyed by heat, alkalinity, and exposure to air. Here's how to preserve your C.

- Buy vegetables in small quantities and eat promptly. Cut your vegetables minimally because more cutting means more vitamin C loss to the air. Keep the skins on.
- Use frozen foods immediately. Plunge them directly into boiling water—don't thaw first.
- Don't use iron or copper pans. They hasten vitamin C breakdown.
- Broil or steam vegetables instead of boiling. If you do boil, do so for as short a time as possible.

Be a spud man. Potatoes and other tubers are respectable vitamin C sources because they retain vitamin C longer than green, leafy vegetables. A new potato, for example, will have 30 milligrams of vitamin C per 100 grams of weight and lose just 70 percent of that in nine months.

Supplement your nutritional income. Don't ignore the benefits of taking vitamin C supplements. "If you lived in a perfect world in a perfect environment eating a perfect diet and had perfect genes, you *might* still benefit from supplements," Dr. Janson says.

Watch out for withdrawal. Researchers have eyeballed a potential pitfall with taking megadoses of vitamin C: addiction. Not like drug addiction, but more like dependence. Your body grows so accustomed to high C levels that it becomes adept at disposing of the excess.

If you suddenly drop to a more moderate amount, your body's disposal system might not adjust fast enough, resulting in a potential deficiency and even scurvy. This is yet another reason not to take megadoses without the guidance of your physician.

Vitamin D

- **Where You Get It:** Fortified milk, fatty fish (herring, kipper, mackerel), liver, egg yolk.

- **What It Does for You:** Increases calcium absorption, aids bone growth and integrity, and promotes sound teeth.

- **What a Man Needs:** Daily Value of 400 international units.

- **Cautions:** Too much causes elevated calcium levels, which may be characterized by low appetite, increased thirst, nausea, vomiting, and weakness. Because vitamin D can be so toxic, do not take more than 600 international units daily unless your doctor prescribes a higher dosage. Too little can soften and deform bones and cause muscle twitching and convulsions.

Vitamin D is a bit of an oddball in the ranks of vitamins and minerals that your body needs to survive. What's special about vitamin D, and what makes it so autonomous?

Simply put, many scientists don't consider vitamin D a vitamin at all. The substance we call vitamin D acts and functions more like a hormone than a vitamin, and by hormone we mean a substance produced by the body for the body. Like other hormones (and vitamin A, another oddball), vitamin D affects you at the cellular level. It does this with its ability to penetrate the inner sanctum of a cell, the nucleus, where it dances with DNA or its protein-based wrapping to make its mark on the body's physiology.

Also unlike its brethren B, C, or E, vitamin D stands alone because it's not an essential nutrient. That doesn't mean that it's unnecessary, mind you; it just means you may not have to add any extra to your diet. As strange as it sounds, no trace of vitamin D need ever cross your lips again—in theory—for you to lead a happy and healthy life. Because the one thing that truly separates vitamin D from its alphabet family is that it's possible for most adults, especially in sunny locales, to get sufficient vitamin D from sunlight exposure.

"If you're working long hours behind a desk, not getting outside and seeing the sunlight, then that's certainly going to be a factor in almost every man's life when it comes to vitamin D," says Dr. Mara Vitolins of the Bowman Gray School of Medicine of Wake Forest University. "Sunlight is what converts those endogenous stores of vitamin D into something you can use."

Seeing the Light

Just how your body uses sunshine to make vitamin D is about as arcane as how the IRS computes your annual standard deduction. Suffice it to say, though, that the four-step process takes about 36 hours and uses the ultraviolet portion of the sun's rays and your own body heat.

In this process, the body first goes to work on a precursor to vitamin D. Oddly enough, the precursor, the raw material from which vitamin D is made, starts out as cholesterol in the liver. It's a fine and often understated example of the human body's "good" uses for cholesterol.

Going through the motions of converting a vitamin D precursor into the real thing takes work, and the body wouldn't go through these motions unless it was important. Indeed, it is. Vitamin D plays a crucial role in bone formation, especially in children, which is why experts suggest that kids get twice as much vitamin D as grown-ups. Even men up to age 24 should get twice as much as the average man age 25 and older.

Considering all the work it does in

keeping you literally standing tall, you need to make sure that you're getting enough vitamin D.

"Because your body can manufacture vitamin D doesn't mean that you should ignore it," Dr. Vitolins says. "I always recommend dairy products. Milk really does do the body good."

Unfortunately, it takes about a quart of milk to give you what you need in any given day. Still, a couple of glasses a day are a good start. Here are other ways that you can play D like a pro.

Let the sun shine. No, this isn't a *Hair* revival. As we said before, sunlight is critical in helping your body synthesize its own vitamin D. Ten minutes of summer sun on your hands and face provide enough exposure for one day, says H. F. DeLuca, Ph.D., chairman of the department of biochemistry at the University of Wisconsin in Madison. If you're dark-skinned, you'll have to prolong your exposure, because dark-pigment skin takes about 3 hours to reach the same level of vitamin D synthesis that fair skin reaches in 30 minutes.

"It depends on where you are in relation to the equator, but in northern climates during the winter, the sun is at such an angle that the right rays don't penetrate the skin to make vitamin D," Dr. DeLuca says. "You can store up quite a bit of vitamin D in your fat cells, so if your diet is good, it will probably last you through winter."

Note that sunlight through a window doesn't count. Glass filters out the rays that you need most.

Don't lay on the lotion. If you're out in the sun, make sure that you cover up with a sunscreen, since too much exposure prematurely wrinkles your skin and possibly puts you at risk for skin cancer. Because sunscreens with a sun-protection factor (SPF) of

The State of Vitamin D

Researchers in Boston have determined the further north you live, the more vitamin D you might need in your diet during certain times of the year. "If you're living in a low-sunlight area during the winter, you could stand outside naked all day and still not make any vitamin D," says Michael F. Holick, M.D., Ph.D., director of the Vitamin D, Skin, and Bone Research Laboratory at Boston University Medical Center.

What do you do if you're Nanook of the North in the winter? Make sure that you get at least 200 IU of vitamin D a day from the food you eat or the supplements you take, if you live in one of the low-sunlight areas below, says Dr. Holick.

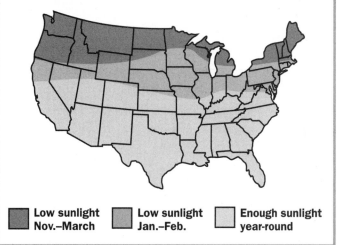

| Low sunlight Nov.–March | Low sunlight Jan.–Feb. | Enough sunlight year-round |

8 or higher stymie vitamin D synthesis, your best bet is to apply sunscreen after enough time has passed for adequate vitamin D production.

Get egg-cited. Egg yolks also are a good source of vitamin D, as are liver, fatty fish, butter, and fortified margarine. That's not to say that you have free rein to mainline these foods. They still may present a risk to your heart's health. But realize that, in moderation, they can help boost your vitamin D levels, Dr. Vitolins says.

Vitamin E

• **Where You Get It:** Salad and cooking oils (except coconut oil), seeds and nuts, wheat germ, asparagus, avocado, beef and organ meats, seafood, apples, carrots, celery.

• **What It Does for You:** Antioxidant powers protect your cells from oxidation. Essential for red blood cells; aids cellular respiration; protects lung tissue from pollution.

• **What a Man Needs:** Daily Value of 30 international units.

• **Cautions:** Deficiency is very rare. Also, it's hard to get too much. (Doses above 300 international units sometimes cause nausea and gastrointestinal problems.) If you are considering taking amounts above 600 international units, discuss this with your doctor first.

Vitamin E is among the most popular of vitamins and, perhaps, the most sensationalized, threatening to topple even the reigning media darling, vitamin C, in the fight for limelight.

But what do you really know about vitamin E other than it's supposed to be pretty good for you? If it weren't for two university researchers and a roomful of frisky laboratory rats, you and the rest of us might not know anything.

It all started in California. The year was 1922. The school, the University of California. Two scientists were working on a piece of lettuce and wheat germ. That is, they were studying it—it was laboratory time, not lunchtime. The scientists were trying to isolate a nutritional substance from lettuce and wheat germ that helped rats reproduce. Eventually, the intrepid duo struck gold. Or, more precisely, they struck upon a gold-colored, fat-soluble chemical, which they promptly named Factor X. Two years later, researchers at the University of Arkansas renamed Factor X vitamin E, presumably because Factor X sounded like a bad science fiction flick.

It wasn't until 12 years later that anyone knew anything more about the substance. In 1936, those wily California researchers said "lettuce experiment more" and got their X in gear. Herbert McLean Evans, along with some new co-workers, isolated a crystalline substance from wheat germ oil. Evans dubbed this new substance *tocopherol*, from the Greek words *tokos*, meaning "offspring," and *pherein*, meaning "to bear." Evans named the substance thus for the role it played in rat procreation, meaning it helped "bring forth offspring" in his whiskered companions.

Thanks to that pioneering groundwork and a lot of modern research, we know today that tocopherol is really a group of substances collectively called vitamin E. In other words, despite what you've been told by the media and that sandal-wearing clerk at the health food store, there is no such thing as vitamin E. In reality, vitamin E is a compound of eight chemical cousins, consisting of the tocopherols, the more active substances, and the tocotrienols, the less active substances. The leader of the pack is alpha-tocopherol, the most biologically active substance and the one commonly considered *the* vitamin E when nothing else is specified. Likewise, alpha-tocopherol is the compound most often reproduced as a synthetic supplement.

In its natural form, vitamin E compounds are yellow viscous oils that are insoluble in water. They also stand up pretty well to light, heat, and acids but are destroyed easily by oxygen and ultraviolet light.

In the body, vitamin E requires bile and fat for proper absorption, most of which takes place in the small intestines, where 20 to 30 percent of vitamin E is whisked away into the body's lymph channels. (Lymph, as you'll recall from seventh-grade science, is a body fluid that contains white blood cells and plays an important role in the immune system.)

Vitamin E storage in the body is generally confined to fatty tissue, the liver, and muscles. Vitamin E excretion takes place almost exclusively through defecation.

Hero of the Heart

You'd think that a vitamin so heavily researched would hold little wonder for a researcher who has seen it all.

Not so.

"The thing I find most fascinating about vitamin E is the fact that vitamin E, a fat-soluble vitamin, might actually slow the development of atherosclerosis," says Dr. Mara Vitolins of the Bowman Gray School of Medicine of Wake Forest University. "In other words, it's interesting to me that a vitamin you get from fats and oils—which can cause hardening of the arteries—might actually help prevent heart problems, which have long been associated with these factors."

Two joint studies looking at more than 127,000 people reported that those who took vitamin E supplements for at least two years had a 40 percent lower risk for heart disease than those who didn't. Another study, this one by Japanese researchers, found that 74 volunteers given 100 milligrams of vitamin E daily showed a definite decreased risk for heart disease, compared to a control group of 73 volunteers taking just 3 milligrams a day.

Experts believe that part of vitamin E's power is the role it plays as an antioxidant in

Know What You're Taking

When it comes to boosting your vitamin E with supplements, make sure that you know what you're getting. And make sure that you're getting the most—for your money and for your health.

Most supplements will be of alpha-tocopherol, the most biologically active of the eight substances collectively known as vitamin E. If your vitamin jar label has a "d-" before "alpha-tocopherol," it means that the vitamin is from natural sources. It also means you paid a little more. A "dl-" before the "alpha-tocopherol" means that it's synthesized and thereby a little less potent. (And less expensive.) "The 'dl-' or 'd-' refers to the chemical structure of alpha-tocopherol," says Dr. Cindy J. Fuller of the University of North Carolina. "In lay terms, there's only one form of the vitamin in d-alpha-tocopherol, and it's the one found in natural sources. The dl type is synthetic, and it comes in eight forms, or isomers, which is where it starts to get confusing."

Does your body care if you're popping a d or dl variation of vitamin E? Probably not, Dr. Fuller says. Moreover, because you'll have to take a little extra of the synthetic form to equal the potency of the natural form, you'll wind up shelling out about the same amount cash-wise for the same effect health-wise.

"This sounds very confusing, but most vitamin E supplements are sold on an international units (IU) basis, so the bottom line is that 400 IU of d equals 400 IU of dl," Dr. Fuller says. "As long as the supplements are sold on an IU basis, you might as well buy the less expensive version."

the body. Antioxidants are substances that neutralize oxidation, the process that causes intercellular breakdown and, perhaps, everything from cancer to the ravages of aging. An antioxidant like vitamin E works by giving up one of its electrons to stabilize a nasty electron-deficient molecule called a free radical.

Free radicals, in their search to become stable, can rob healthy molecules of their electrons, resulting in damage. Vitamin E, as an antioxidant, inhibits oxidation of polyunsaturated fatty acids, Dr. Vitolins says.

Another fascinating thing about vitamin E is the role it plays in helping other antioxidants. Like a vitamin vigilante, vitamin E protects vitamin C, vitamin A, and carotene (along with a few other things) from being oxidized, allowing *them* to perform *their* critical roles unhindered by a free radical ambush.

"This is why most people talk about the 'ACE' vitamins, when they're talking about antioxidants. Vitamins A, C, and E tend to work so well together," says health and fitness consultant Dr. Richard F. Gerson.

Other fascinating facts about vitamin E: include the following

- Research at the University of Arizona College of Medicine's Health Sciences Center in Tucson has found that vitamin E might reduce age-associated damage in both the immune and central nervous systems. "The results suggest that vitamin E, and possibly other antioxidants, may reduce damage associated with aging," says Marguerite Kay, M.D., professor of microbiology, immunology, and medicine at the university and the study's lead investigator.
- Researchers think that vitamin E might prevent lung damage associated with smoking. One study of 83 male smokers and 65 nonsmoking men found that, while both groups had about the same levels of vitamin E in their blood, the smokers' bodies showed an increased

Ease Muscles with E

Do grueling workouts have you down? Some promising research suggests that you'll spring back faster by taking vitamin E and other antioxidants. While dietary antioxidant supplements, like E or C, have no proven benefit for healthy, young athletes, older "weekend warriors" like yourself might see a noticeable benefit by sneaking a little extra antioxidant power after exercise.

Delayed-onset muscle soreness, or DOMS, is a condition most of us know too well. We spend our days jockeying a desk and then play a weekend game of touch football, only to find ourselves feeling stiff as a board Monday morning. That's because exercise can cause microscopic tears in muscles unaccustomed to such overexertion.

Some experts theorize that this muscle mayhem may last for a couple of days because there's a surge of free-

need for E, apparently to make up for the damage that smoking was causing their lungs.

- One Harvard study tracking 40,000 male health professionals over four years found that those with diets highest in vitamin E developed 36 percent fewer cases of heart disease than those who consumed the least amount of vitamin E. Moreover, those who took supplements of 100 international units a day for at least two years were 37 percent less likely to develop heart disease than those who took no supplements.

Eat Your Fill

Getting the vitamin E you need is pretty easy. It starts with eating a healthy diet in general, but you can supersize your E levels with a little help.

radical activity in the muscles themselves. Antioxidants might help neutralize those minuscule thugs, thus minimizing the pain and damage.

One study from the Noll Physiological Research Center at Pennsylvania State University in University Park found that vitamin E supplements in older exercisers increased their ability to bounce back from DOMS. This effect was not found in younger, active adults, or in distance athletes, who seem to have a well-developed antioxidant system to begin with.

So if you feel like a hit-and-run case on Monday because of the game on Saturday, your best bet is to get on a regular exercise routine. That way your body will be primed for action all the time.

Barring that, ask your doctor about taking a little extra vitamin E to relieve muscle aches and pains in the meantime.

Cut your losses. A lot of your food's natural vitamin E is gone before it ever gets to you. That's because processing and packaging destroy E in many ways. Milling grain to convert whole wheat to white flour, for example, removes 80 percent of the grain's vitamin E. Canning causes losses of 41 to 65 percent in meats and vegetables, and roasting nuts robs them of up to 80 percent of their vitamin E.

You may not have any control over what the processing and manufacturing companies do, but you can cut your own losses by not deep-frying your food. Deep-frying destroys 32 to 75 percent of a food's E.

Chip in for extra E. Here's good news for every man alive: Potato chips are an excellent source of E, but know that your chips will lose up to 70 percent or more if stored for over a month. (But that's still no reason to eat them all at once.)

Clean up smog-E situations. Life in the concrete jungle is hell. You not only have to watch out for errant taxicabs and wayward muggers, you have to watch what you breathe, too. Vitamin E helps do that for you. Studies show that vitamin E protects lung tissue from nasty things in the air, like nitrogen dioxide, which can oxidize cells in your lungs. It's not clear whether E is good against pollution in general, but it shows promise.

Defend against diabetes. Vitamin E might be a friend in warding off adult-onset diabetes. One study from Finland looked at almost 1,000 men ages 42 to 60, none of whom had diabetes.

Four years later, the men were again evaluated, and researchers found that 45 developed diabetes within that time, mostly those with the lowest blood levels of vitamin E. In fact, below-average levels of E indicated a 400 percent increase in risk to develop diabetes, compared to normal levels.

Don't mistake E for "erotic." Remember those pioneering studies we told you about? The ones where early researchers looked for vitamin E because it enhanced procreation in laboratory rats? Unless you have a tail and long whiskers and love cheese, don't think about taking vitamin E to supercharge your sex life. There's a mistaken belief that vitamin E is a sex vitamin and that it will reduce sterility and increase potency. It will—for rodents.

E-rase scars. Vitamin E's positive effects on cells may help when it comes to healing scars, too.

In one study of people ranging from age 18 to 63, researchers added vitamin E to silicone gel sheets that were used to treat scars. Ninety-five percent of the 40 people who got E showed 50 percent improvement after eight weeks, compared to the same level of improvement in 75 percent of the 40 patients who didn't get vitamin E.

Vitamin K

• **Where You Get It:** Green tea, turnip greens, broccoli, lettuce, cabbage, spinach, liver, asparagus, bacon, coffee, cheese.

• **What It Does for You:** Controls blood coagulation; essential for synthesizing liver proteins that control clotting.

• **What a Man Needs:** Daily Value of 80 micrograms.

• **Cautions:** Too little results in delayed blood clotting and hemorrhagic disease in newborn infants. Natural forms of vitamin K are seemingly nontoxic, but synthetic versions have caused jaundice when given in doses of more than 5 milligrams a day.

Like many other vitamins, vitamin K is actually one name representing several compounds, all of which are vital to human life. The compounds, known as the quinones, help create blood clotting substances manufactured in the liver.

Vitamin K was discovered in the 1930s by Danish biochemist Carl Peter Hendrick Dam of the University of Copenhagen, who noticed that certain diets in baby chicks caused lethal and uncontrollable hemorrhages. In 1935, Dam named the substance he believed was responsible for controlling clotting the *Koagulation* vitamin, from the Danish word for coagulation. The name later was shortened to vitamin K, and Dam received a Nobel prize in physiology and medicine in 1943 for his discovery.

Natural vitamin K comes in the form of a light yellow oil. Synthetically, it's a yellow crystalline powder. Strangely, clotting seems to be the only use science has identified for vitamin K. Not that it does the job single-handedly—at least 13 different substances are involved in blood clotting. But vitamin K helps create at least 4 of those substances, including the biggie, prothrombin, which is created in the liver as a precursor to thrombin, the material that actually spins the clot, so to speak.

Here's how to be A-OK.

Reach for fresh food. Fresh food is the best source for vitamin K. Frozen foods tend to be lacking. Stick to the produce aisle when you're shopping for fresh broccoli, spinach, and asparagus.

Go for goodness in the gut. Vitamin K also comes from naturally occurring bacteria in your intestine. Unfortunately, the amount produced in the gut isn't enough to meet all your needs, so don't neglect a nutritious diet. (Interestingly, newborn babies are born without intestinal flora. They're given a 1-milligram shot of vitamin K at birth.)

Check with your doctor if you're taking anticoagulants. Sometimes a physician will prescribe an anticoagulant to keep a patient's blood from clotting. There are cases on record where a vitamin K–rich diet was enough to counteract the effect of the medication. Ask your doctor if your vitamin K intake should be a concern if you're ever prescribed an anticoagulant.

But don't cut the K from your diet arbitrarily. And be wary if your doctor suggests that you do cut the K, says John W. Suttie, Ph.D., professor and chairman of nutritional science at the University of Wisconsin in Madison.

The key, says Dr. Suttie, is to keep your levels of vitamin K consistent so that the medication dosage can be prescribed with that consistent K level in mind.

Don't cut all the fat. As far as vitamin K is concerned, a little fat is a good thing. And a little goes a long way. The body absorbs vitamin K only when there's a bit of dietary fat present, so if you're eating K-consciously, make sure that you include a little fat to make it worth your while. A little means a dollop of oil-based dressing on your spinach salad, not drenching it with dressing or scarfing down a half-loaf of heavily buttered bread.

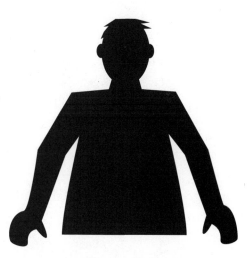

Part Three

Making Mineral Deposits

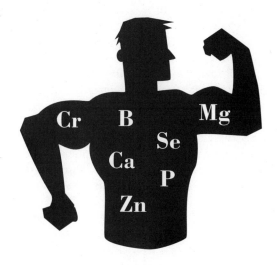

Boron

- **Where You Get It:** Wine, prunes, dates, raisins, honey.

- **What It Does for You:** Works with calcium, magnesium, and vitamin D to prevent bone loss. May help you stay more alert.

- **What a Man Needs:** There is no Daily Value, but 1 to 2 milligrams a day is safe and possibly advantageous.

- **Cautions:** Contrary to popular opinion, boron does not help build muscle. If you see it advertised as a strength-building supplement, then the company is misleading you.

Boron is one of the most recent additions to the list of possible essential mineral elements, because researchers have discovered that it enhances the body's ability to use calcium, which may help maintain better bone health.

"We can't say that boron is an essential mineral, because a specific biochemical effect hasn't been discovered yet," says Forrest Nielsen, Ph.D., director of the U.S. Department of Agriculture–Agricultural Research Service Grand Forks Human Nutrition Research Center in North Dakota. "But it does seem that boron makes vitamin D and other bone-improving hormones and minerals more efficient."

Oddly enough, boron's history began as a food preservative in the 1870s, when it was used in the form of borax and boric acid. At first considered innocuous, countries actually began to outlaw its addition to foods when it was found that dosages of 500 milligrams a day caused appetite disturbances. Today, researchers understand that boron is beneficial, if not essential, to humans.

Its main benefit seems to be maximizing the body's use of calcium and magnesium. This is good news for those people at risk for osteoporosis.

Just as important, boron seems to play a role in brain function. "When people who normally eat low-boron diets supplemented with 3 milligrams a day, they report feeling more mentally alert," says Dr. Nielsen. "Motor function is improved." In fact, the low-boron diets seem to cause electrical changes in the brain that are similar to those found in people with malnutrition. There is evidence that boron may play a role in cognition, he says.

Unfortunately, boron has been misrepresented in the press as a muscle-building mineral, says Dr. Nielsen. "It's hogwash," he adds. "In 1987 I reported that when postmenopausal women were given a boron supplement, there was a slight increase in testosterone, but it was a small increase up to normal levels for women. I've since looked at men in the other studies, and it had no effect on testosterone. In terms of boron being a muscle-builder, it's bunk."

Because boron is an essential nutrient for plants, you can find it in numerous foods, such as fresh fruits and nuts. The western United States has more boron in its water than the eastern states. One glass of wine has slightly less than 1 milligram of boron. Your body absorbs boron easily, and no other mineral seems to counteract the work that it does.

The average American seems to consume 0.5 to 3.1 milligrams a day through food and water. However, since boron has yet to be labeled essential, you won't find it in all multivitamin/mineral supplements. And if you do find it in a multi, the amount will be small, such as the 150 micrograms found in Centrum.

"I recommend a daily intake of 1 to 2 milligrams," says Dr. Nielsen. "I am concerned about that small percentage of the population that gets less than 0.5 milligram a day."

Boron is safe up to 10 milligrams a day, says Dr. Nielsen, but there doesn't seem to be any reason to supplement to those numbers.

Calcium

- ***Where You Get It:*** Cheese, molasses, yogurt, beans, bread.

- ***What It Does for You:*** Builds strong teeth and bones and stimulates nerve impulses (magnesium relaxes them).

- ***What a Man Needs:*** Daily Value of 1,000 milligrams.

- ***Cautions:*** Taking more than 2,000 milligrams a day may cause constipation and kidney stones and inhibit zinc and iron absorption. Calcium supplements can cause bloating, gas, and confusion, especially in older men. When taken together, calcium and tetracycline form an insoluble chemical complex that impairs both mineral and drug absorption.

Sometime after you turn 30, you start to lose a little backbone with each passing year. That's not a commentary on the psychological state of aging men. It's a medical fact.

As you age, you naturally lose bone mass. Your best defense is to make sure that you get enough calcium in your diet. "Aside from calcium, bone consists of high levels of phosphorus and a good quantity of magnesium as well as trace elements of zinc" says Mona Calvo, Ph.D., a member of the clinical research and review staff for the Food and Drug Administration in Washington, D.C. "And vitamin D must be present for the body to efficiently absorb calcium."

In fact, adults usually absorb only 20 to 30 percent of the calcium they consume. But here's what you really need to know: Your body has a complex mechanism to maintain sufficient calcium levels in your blood, which is essential to keep muscles and nerves healthy.

To keep this level of calcium constant, the body either takes calcium from the bone and puts it into the blood or absorbs calcium from the blood and puts it into the bone.

If you don't get enough calcium in your diet, your body pulls the mineral from the calcium reserves in your bones, weakening them. As you get older, if you don't eat enough calcium, your body gradually takes more calcium from your bones than it puts in them. Left unchecked, that gradual erosion can lead to osteoporosis, a degenerative disease in which the bones become so fragile that they break in response to even slight trauma. You may have seen elderly men walking around in a stooped position. That's because some of the vertebrae in the spine have collapsed or broken, and this causes the spine to curve.

Although it occurs much later in life in men than it does in women, whenever you lose height, it usually means that you have experienced a collapsed vertebra as a result of bone loss in the spine. This loss happens over a long period of time. As men begin to live longer, osteoporosis will become a greater health concern.

Currently, severe osteoporosis afflicts only 15 percent of men before age 85. However, research suggests that half of us are getting less than 800 milligrams of calcium a day, well under the 1,000 milligrams recommended. And what a difference a few hundred milligrams can make. Robert Heaney, M.D., professor of medicine at Creighton University in Omaha, Nebraska, and a leading calcium expert, estimates that getting enough calcium could prevent as many as half of all osteoporotic fractures.

Aside from creating strong teeth and bones, calcium is critical for the proper functioning of other organ systems, such as muscle contraction and blood clotting. So a shortage of calcium will prevent you from attaining optimal health in other ways, too.

Even if you do get enough calcium in your diet, caffeine, alcohol, and cigarette smoke can contribute to the body's loss of calcium. On the other hand, weight-bearing exercise, such as walking or running, will help the bones maintain their density over the years.

A Man's Plan

So, what should your calcium plan be? Milk and other foods rich in calcium and vitamin D, and foods fortified with calcium, Dr. Calvo says. "Not only is milk rich in calcium but also the vitamin D and protein in milk facilitate absorption," she says. You can also choose cheese and other low-fat dairy foods to get calcium.

Today, manufacturers are adding calcium to a variety of foods. Orange juice, for example, often has it. "It's very hard to keep calcium in a solution. Citrus juice is actually a good medium, but make sure you that shake it up and drink it fairly quickly," says Dr. Calvo. Why? So that the calcium doesn't settle to the bottom of the container. The same is true for fortified lactose-free milk drinks, such as Lactaid.

Other products with added calcium include some cereals, corn tortillas, and English muffins. Green vegetables such as kale, broccoli, and Chinese cabbage (bok choy) are also good sources of naturally available calcium.

That doesn't mean, however, that you can stop drinking your milk. "Orange juice doesn't give you vitamin D, and many people in the United States don't get enough D," says Dr. Calvo. "African-Americans and others with darker skin can't always synthesize enough vitamin D (the sunshine vitamin), especially during the winter months when there's little sunshine available." That's why milk is also important to most adults.

Supplementing Your Stores

If you just don't eat any type of dairy product, then you may want to consider taking calcium supplements. And if you head to the store for calcium supplements, you'll find lots to choose from. But you won't find a considerable amount in most multivitamins because calcium is a bulky mineral and is hard to fit in a multivitamin tablet that is small enough to swallow.

Calcium supplements come from a variety of original, natural sources, including oyster shells, ground bone, and limestone. Manufacturers can purify these to varying degrees or combine them with other compounds such as citrate or gluconate. Your body absorbs and uses these various types of calcium supplements differently, so you need to choose wisely. Based on limited research, it seems that most healthy people absorb calcium equally well from calcium supplements that are a combination of amino acids bonded with calcium, calcium phosphate dibasic, or calcium acetate, carbonate, citrate, gluconate, or lactate. People don't absorb calcium as well from oyster shell calcium fortified with inorganic magnesium, from chelated calcium-magnesium combinations, calcium carbonate fortified with vitamins and iron, or a mixture of calcium and magnesium carbonates.

To aid absorption, calcium citrate should be taken on an empty stomach, while another popular form, calcium carbonate, is best taken with food.

"Your calcium tablet may not have the other things required for proper calcium absorption," says Dr. Calvo. Some people take combined calcium and vitamin D products. Other products contain essential trace minerals good for bones, such as magnesium and zinc. Some supplements have side effects, so if your stomach is queasy after taking one, consider drinking a glass or two (8 ounces each) of milk.

Some men are concerned that calcium supplements may cause kidney stones. Kidney stones affect more men than women for reasons that are not entirely clear. We do know that those who are prone to form and pass stones may also hyper-absorb calcium. Most men don't find out they are hyper-absorbers of calcium until they pass a stone. If kidney stones run in your family, talk to your doctor about calcium intake; but chances are that he'll tell you to at least keep it to the Daily Value of 1,000 milligrams.

Chromium

• **Where You Get It:** Blackstrap molasses, apple peels, beer.

• **What It Does for You:** Acts cooperatively with other substances to control insulin and certain enzymes.

• **What a Man Needs:** Daily Value of 120 micrograms.

• **Cautions:** Do not supplement above 200 micrograms unless you are under your doctor's supervision. Also, if you are diabetic, do not supplement with chromium without doctor supervision, since high intakes of it can cause your blood sugar levels to drop dangerously low.

Why do those chrome fenders shine so? Because of chromium, a mineral that derives its name from the Greek word *chroma*, meaning "multicolored." And that same mineral can help keep you shining in good health.

Most important to men is chromium's role as a component of glucose tolerance factor (GTF), a hormonelike agent that also contains niacin and some amino acids. GTF enters the blood when there is an increase of insulin in the bloodstream. It enhances the effect of insulin by making the sugars pass more easily into the cells. If there isn't enough GTF in the system, the sugars may stay in the blood, which can lead to diabetes.

Chromium levels in the body decline with age, and the ability to convert chromium to GTF may also decline with age and could be one of the explanations for adult-onset diabetes. The average diet with plenty of refined flour and sugar also leaves people with lots of sugar to process but very little chromium to help get the job done.

"If you eat a whole grain, you get chromium. But when grain is processed to remove the fiber and the bran, the chromium is also removed," says Cathy Kapica, R.D., Ph.D., associate professor of nutrition and clinical dietetics at Finch University of Health Sciences/Chicago Medical School. "Those processed grains use up the chromium in your body without replacing it, so over the years, you can develop a chromium deficiency that may mimic diabetes."

Although the Daily Value for chromium is 120 micrograms, the U.S. Department of Agriculture (USDA) estimates that most adults get only about 33 micrograms of chromium every day in their diets. Many multivitamin/mineral supplements include chromium, but some contain less than the Daily Value.

Chromium's reputation as a carbohydrate burner has left many weight lifters with the mistaken belief that chromium burns fat and builds muscle and strength. Chromium picolinate is one of the hottest supplements on the market.

"Studies have shown that we absorb only about 1 percent of the chromium that we consume, and chromium picolinate is one of the best absorbed of the different types of chromium," says Dr. Forrest Nielsen of the USDA–Agricultural Research Service Grand Forks Human Nutrition Research Center.

But, adds Dr. Nielsen, you only see an increase in chromium's effectiveness if you have a deficiency. "Anything above an adequate intake won't help you. It's a fairly ineffective supplement for bodybuilding, even though it's sold as a supplement to increase muscle mass." He believes that the amount in a typical multivitamin is more than enough, especially if it's complementing a diet containing whole grains.

"You can take too much chromium; 200 micrograms a day would be the maximum amount," adds Dr. Kapica. "And people who are taking large amounts of supplements aren't helping themselves as much as they would be if they were eating more whole grains and less refined flour and sugar."

Iron

• **Where to Get It:** Meat, fortified cereals consumed with orange juice.

• **What It Does for You:** Makes your blood nice and red. Aids in the transportation of oxygen throughout the body.

• **What a Man Needs:** Daily Value of 18 milligrams.

• **Cautions:** Too much iron has been linked to higher risk of heart disease and cancer in men. Iron supplements are the leading cause of pediatric death from poisoning. So if you have supplements with iron in the house, keep them away from children. A fatal dose of iron for a toddler can be as little as 600 milligrams, which is how much iron you might find in as few as four iron supplement tablets.

Take a vat of cold water and plunge a fire-hot sword into it. Let the water cool. Drink up. You have just cured yourself of anemia, ancient Greek–style. While it may be one of the more romantic ways to fight a deficiency disease, sword dipping isn't always reliable. These days we have less poetic but more effective solutions.

"Actually, the truth is that few men, if any, need more iron," says David Meyers, M.D., professor of internal medicine and preventive medicine at University of Kansas School of Medicine in Kansas City. "In fact, almost all men need less iron than they are consuming."

Studies have begun to show that heart disease, the number one killer of men, may somehow be linked to high iron levels in men. "Women only have 30 to 50 percent of the rate of arteriosclerosis as men do, and they get it 10

to 15 years later," says Dr. Meyers. "We have traditionally ascribed that protection to the presence of estrogen, but studies have shown that it isn't just estrogen that seems to protect women, but their periods. Maybe women get less heart disease because they lose iron every month."

This, however, is just a hypothesis, says Janet Hunt, R.D., Ph.D., research nutrition scientist for the U.S. Department of Agriculture–Agricultural Research Service Grand Forks Human Nutrition Research Center in North Dakota. "We haven't seen proof yet. In the studies conducted so far, persons with heart disease and high iron stores may have been different in other important ways that were not even identified. It would be useful to do a long-term study looking at men who are otherwise similar, but with some who are instructed to donate blood and some who aren't, to see if there's a difference in their rates of heart disease."

Although it is controversial whether high iron stores lead to heart disease, Dr. Hunt and some other researchers think that iron released from damaged tissue, as occurs after a heart attack, can cause oxidative injury. That damage can be prevented by giving patients iron-binding compounds along with drugs that help dissolve clots. But scientists do not agree whether iron can do similar oxidative damage in uninjured tissues. "In normal tissues," says Dr. Hunt, "iron is bound by proteins that make it quite unavailable to participate in damaging chemical reactions."

Even if high iron stores are determined to increase oxidative damage and heart disease, the real problem may lie in relating iron stores to dietary iron. In large surveys, iron supplement users do not have higher iron stores. In controlled studies, attempts to increase the absorption of iron with ascorbic acid supplements or high-meat diets have not increased iron stores after several weeks or even months. Iron stores may be mainly controlled by genetic factors. "Although it is quite clear that iron stores are reduced by blood loss, and that iron supplements correct low iron stores, it is not clear whether high iron intakes increase normal iron stores beyond a biological 'set point,'" says Dr. Hunt. "In fact, the body appears to be able to adjust quite well to greatly increase or decrease the amount of iron absorbed.

Too Much, Not Enough

Still, many researchers believe that iron deficiency is rare in American men and that they are more likely to have too much rather than too little iron. This is, in part, because of the amount of iron-fortified foods that men eat and because the body has no way of ridding itself of excess iron once it has been absorbed by the body, except through blood loss.

So, what does a man need when it comes to iron? The first step is to know where you stand.

"Iron is currently measured in most first-level blood tests," says Lisa Ruml, M.D., assistant professor of medicine at the University of Texas Southwestern Medical Center at Dallas, "though this may change with new Medicare rules. A better test of a person's iron supply, though, is a measurement of ferritin, which is the storage form of iron. So when you go for a physical, ask the doctor to check your iron level. There are lots of things you can do whether he says it's low or high."

Iron absorption levels change radically based on the amounts you have stored in your body. The less iron you have, the more you'll absorb from a meal, while the more iron you have, the less you'll absorb from your diet. Anemia is diagnosed by looking at the hemoglobin value, which is where iron is contained in the red blood cells. In most laboratories, anemia is defined as a hemoglobin value of less than 14 grams per deciliter for men. It is very unlikely that taking an iron supplement will increase your hemoglobin to above normal, but if it does, you may have a condition that makes it difficult for you to use the iron properly and your physician may need to evaluate you further, says Dr. Ruml.

There are two forms of iron in food: heme iron and nonheme iron. "Heme iron is present in red blood cells and in muscles," Dr. Hunt says. "You can find it in meat, poultry, and fish but not in milk, eggs, vegetables, or grains." Heme iron is more easily absorbed by the body.

"All the rest is called nonheme iron," Dr. Hunt says. This includes cereals, fruits, grains, vegetables, and beans. "Nonheme iron is more susceptible to the effects of other foods." The presence of phytic acids in cereal and tannins in tea can block the absorption of iron. Your body absorbs 25 percent of the heme iron available from food, but less than 10 percent of the nonheme iron that is in food. Despite the difference in absorption, both irons are equally beneficial to the body.

"There are a number of things that can decrease your absorption of iron," Dr. Hunt says. "Take in too much copper, calcium, phosphorus, manganese, or zinc and your absorption will be compromised."

If your iron levels are low, have some orange juice along with your steak. (The presence of vitamin C when you eat iron-rich foods will increase your absorption, says Dr. Ruml.) Also, Cream of Wheat is a good source, providing nearly 100 percent of the Recommended Dietary Allowance of iron for men.

These dietary changes can raise or lower the amount of iron your body absorbs over the short term. However, long-term studies of several weeks or months have not found differences in iron stores by following these eating patterns, Dr. Hunt says.

Here are some things you can do if your iron level is high.

Drink tea. "Tannic acid decreases iron stores by interfering with absorption," Dr. Ruml says. Coffee also contains tannic acid.

Supplement smartly. If you take a multivitamin, make sure that you get one without iron.

Eat a salad with your steak. The presence of fiber will decrease the amount of iron that you absorb from a meal. Keep in mind, though, that it is unusual to have high iron stores unless you have a medical condition that predisposes you to it.

Magnesium

• **Where You Get It:** Meats; green, leafy vegetables; brown rice; legumes; nuts; whole grains.

• **What It Does for You:** Helps form bones and teeth. Relaxes nerve impulses that cause muscles to flex (calcium stimulates them) and is essential for cellular metabolism and energy production.

• **What a Man Needs:** Daily Value of 400 milligrams.

• **Cautions:** Overuse of magnesium supplements, antacids, or laxatives can cause magnesium buildup in those with poor kidney function, which can lead to slowed breathing, coma, and sometimes death. Always check with your doctor before taking supplemental magnesium if you have kidney or heart problems.

Although the Romans used magnesia alba (white magnesium salts from the Magnesia district of Greece) to cure many ailments, the element magnesium wasn't isolated until 1808. Today it is recognized as an essential mineral that is second only to potassium in terms of concentration within individual cells of the body.

"Magnesium helps the muscle tone of the heart," says Dr. Lisa Ruml of the University of Texas Southwestern Medical Center at Dallas. "It's very important for all muscle function, and if you're low in magnesium, it's harder to control blood pressure."

In fact, when a researcher at the University of North Carolina in Chapel Hill reviewed years of magnesium studies, she found ample evidence that stress—both physical and emotional—can increase the body's need for magnesium. The hormones catecholamine and corticosteroid are released during stressful episodes and can cause the heart muscle to lose some of its stored magnesium. In turn, a high magnesium level may help fight the strains of stress.

"Although it's not easy to become chronically deficient in magnesium, I think that magnesium is worth using as a supplement," Dr. Ruml advises. Aside from blood pressure problems, low magnesium levels can, over time, rob your bones of vital minerals, leaving them porous and weakened.

You can find 100 milligrams of magnesium in many multivitamin/mineral supplements. But you also can get a supplement of magnesium alone or with its related bone-building nutrients, such as calcium and zinc. Although the Daily Value is 400 milligrams, most men only get about 330 milligrams each day.

"When magnesium is low, the parathyroid gland doesn't work well, and that's what processes vitamin D to better absorb calcium," Dr. Ruml says. "In other words, you can have trouble conserving your calcium in the presence of low magnesium." In fact, when magnesium intake is extremely low, calcium is sometimes deposited in the soft tissues, leading to calcified lesions.

Supplementation may be particularly important because of the link between magnesium and calcium. Magnesium relaxes nerve impulses and muscle contraction, while calcium stimulates them. The two must be in balance to allow the body to function at optimum levels.

Picking the right magnesium supplement may save you a lot of time in the bathroom. Dose for dose, magnesium gluconate causes one-third the amount of diarrhea of magnesium oxide and one-half the frequency of diarrhea of magnesium chloride, says Herbert C. Mansmann Jr., M.D., professor of pediatrics and associate professor of medicine at Jefferson Medical College of Thomas Jefferson University in Philadelphia.

Molybdenum

• *Where You Get It:* Milk, lima beans, spinach, liver, breads, cereals.

• *What It Does for You:* As a component of three different enzymes, it's involved in the metabolism of nucleic acids (DNA and RNA), iron, and food into energy. Helps break down toxic buildups of sulfites in the body. May help prevent cavities.

• *What a Man Needs:* Daily Value of 75 micrograms.

• *Cautions:* Deficiencies rarely happen unless there is an excess of copper or sulfate in the body. Toxicity is also rare, but high concentrations of molybdenum in the environment can cause symptoms of diarrhea, slow growth, and anemia.

With a name like molybdenum, you've got to be tough. And it is. The adult body has about 9 milligrams of molybdenum (pronounced mo-LIB-duh-num) spread fairly evenly throughout it. Even when intake was lowered to 25 micrograms per day—just one-third of the Daily Value—levels of this hardy mineral in the body remained steady, according to a study conducted by the U.S. Department of Agriculture (USDA).

"No natural deficiency of molybdenum in humans has ever been described," says Dr. Forrest Nielsen of the USDA–Agricultural Research Service Grand Forks Human Nutrition Research Center. "And toxicity is also rare in humans, although it is more common in cows who graze on land rich in molybdenum."

Some multivitamin/mineral tablets now contain molybdenum. Up to 250 micrograms of molybdenum a day is estimated by the U.S. National Research Council to be safe and adequate, but there's no reason to take that much. It isn't a mineral that you even need in a supplement, Dr. Nielsen says. The average American diet includes about 93 micrograms a day, well within the recommended limits. However, the body easily rids itself of excess amounts, so don't worry if you see it listed on a supplement label. If you use a multivitamin/mineral that contains molybdenum, make sure that it has no more than 250 micrograms, says Dr. Nielsen.

Amounts higher than 500 micrograms of molybdenum can interfere with your body's metabolism of copper and also can lead to symptoms of gout. On the other hand, too much copper, tungsten, or sulfate can drain the body of molybdenum. This deficiency scenario has only been seen in animals.

"Molybdenum seems to help the body rid itself of the potentially dangerous effects of sulfites and other toxins," Dr. Nielsen says. "We are starting to see evidence that molybdenum may have some antioxidant properties because it fights foreign compounds or drugs that come into the body. If molybdenum isn't there to help your body metabolize them, they can cause cancer, for example. Molybdenum seems to be involved in the detoxification of compounds."

Molybdenum is part of sulfite oxidase, an enzyme that helps the body detoxify sulfites, compounds found in protein foods and used as chemical preservatives in some foods and drugs. People who can't break down sulfites have toxic buildups of this chemical in their bodies, says Judith Turnlund, R.D., Ph.D., of the U.S. Department of Agriculture Western Human Nutrition Research Center in San Francisco.

Some people are supersensitive to the sulfites used as additives, developing asthma and other life-threatening breathing problems.

Molybdenum also is part of two other enzymes: xanthine oxidase and aldehyde oxidase. Both are involved in the body's production of genetic material and proteins. Xanthine oxidase also helps the body produce uric acid, an important waste product.

Phosphorus

• **Where You Get It:** Milk, cereal, meat.

• **What It Does for You:** Helps form bones and teeth, builds muscle, and is involved in almost all metabolic actions in the body.

• **What a Man Needs:** Daily Value of 1,000 milligrams.

• **Cautions:** There is no known toxicity for phosphorus, but too much can cause a deficiency of calcium in the blood.

Phosphorus is the second most abundant mineral in our body, behind calcium. Unlike calcium, phosphorus is naturally found in the majority of foods. It's also available in the beverage section of any grocery store. However, it makes a huge difference whether you get your phosphorus from a can of soda or a glass of milk. And the reason is...calcium.

"There is a constant balancing act going on in your blood and bones to keep calcium and phosphorus in balance," says Dr. Mona Calvo of the Food and Drug Administration.

The ideal phosphorus-to-calcium ratio (milligrams to milligrams) is 1 to 1, says Dr. Calvo, because the Daily Value for both calcium and phosphorus is the same—1,000 milligrams. You can find a level close to the ideal ratio in a glass of milk.

But drink a can of cola and all you get is phosphorus, and no calcium. Phosphoric acid is used to hold the carbonation in colas and some root beers.

"Phosphorus works with calcium, the most abundant mineral in our bodies, to build bone," Dr. Calvo says. When it isn't busy creating bone, phosphorus is part of many components of the cells like adenosine triphos-phate, which is the key compound that stores energy and operates in metabolism. It also functions in almost every other metabolic pathway in the body.

Intake estimates show that while most men consume more than the recommended amount of phosphorus, they sometimes don't get enough calcium.

And according to some studies, when that phosphorus-to-calcium ratio is thrown out of whack, it may lead to decreases in bone mass. More research needs to be done, however, in order to establish this fact in humans.

"Adding to this problem, I believe, is the underreporting of phosphorus levels," Dr. Calvo says. "The more processed foods you eat, the more phosphorus you're getting. It is not required to include phosphorus levels in nutrition labels. Because phosphorus food additives are so useful and serve many functions to improve the food supply, it's almost impossible to avoid getting the Daily Value. The same is not true for calcium.

"You need a number of different minerals to help your bones stay strong," Dr. Calvo says. You can find many of these in a glass of milk rather than a pill.

Some food sources with good ratios of calcium to phosphorus include apples, broccoli, carrots, corn, ground beef, roasted turkey, strawberries, and tuna. Dairy products are the best sources overall, Dr. Calvo says.

The phosphorus in meats and dairy foods is more bioavailable than the phosphorus found in cereals, fruits, and vegetables. Unlike calcium, phosphorus is very efficiently absorbed.

Although aluminum hydroxide, which is the main ingredient in a number of antacids, can interfere with absorption, deficiencies of phosphorus are almost unheard of.

"At this point phosphorus seems to be everywhere in the food supply," Dr. Calvo says. "And that's more of a problem than any deficiency issue."

Potassium

- **Where You Get It:** Dried fruits, most raw vegetables, citrus fruits, molasses, sunflower seeds.

- **What It Does for You:** Helps keep blood pressure down and aids muscle contraction, healthy electrical activity in the heart, and rapid transmission of nerve impulses throughout the body.

- **What a Man Needs:** Daily Value of 3,500 milligrams.

- **Cautions:** Don't supplement without a physician's consent if you have kidney problems or diabetes or are taking digitalis, some diuretics, or blood pressure medication. A normal kidney will excrete any excess potassium that the body doesn't need, so it is not necessary to take large amounts of potassium. A normal, balanced diet is more than adequate for most people.

Bouncers just don't get the respect they deserve. If some jerk is causing trouble in your favorite watering hole, chances are that you're grateful if there's a bouncer around to give him the old heave-ho. Potassium is one of your body's "bouncers." And chances are that you don't give it the respect it deserves.

If you're scarfing down too much sodium every day—and most of us are—potassium helps give it the bum's rush from your body and flushes out excess fluid from your blood. And along with sodium, magnesium, and calcium, potassium helps keep your heart beating in time like the drummer on your favorite jukebox tune. If these minerals are not in balance, the blood vessels may become stiff, creating high blood pressure. "One of the first things you may notice, though, if you are low in potassium, is muscle weakness or a loss of stamina overall," says Dr. Lisa Ruml of the University of Texas Southwestern Medical Center at Dallas.

So here's the problem: Most of us have thrown that delicate balance way out of whack. While the Daily Value for potassium is 3,500 milligrams, we get an average of about 2,500 milligrams a day. Meanwhile, the Daily Value for sodium is 2,400 milligrams, but we consume anywhere from 2,000 to 6,000 milligrams daily.

"Most men need to cut down on sodium and increase their intake of natural potassium, such as dried fruits or citrus fruits and bananas," says Dr. Ruml. "We used to think that you just needed to watch sodium to control high blood pressure, but now we know that potassium is also important."

This is especially true for African-American men, whose diets tend to be lower in potassium than White men and who also have higher rates of high blood pressure. Researchers gave 43 African-American men potassium supplements (3,120 milligrams a day) and another 43 placebos. The men who took the potassium had an average drop in their blood pressures of 6.9 points. The men who took placebos showed no changes.

It's rare that anyone will suffer from a potassium-deficiency disease, Dr. Ruml says, but when you're sick with the flu or anything that upsets your digestion, you might need more potassium, since vomiting and diarrhea can deplete your potassium reserves. The main symptom of potassium deficiency is weakness.

"When a person goes to the doctor complaining of fatigue, weakness, or a lack of stamina, his doctor will look at the potassium and calcium levels in his blood because these electrolytes control the work that muscles do," Dr. Ruml says.

Electrolytes, which include sodium and potassium, dissolve in water. Potassium, calcium, and magnesium live within cells, while sodium sets up house mainly in the bloodstream. While only sodium and potassium are electrolytes, all four minerals work with muscles. Potassium and magnesium relax muscles, while sodium and calcium contract them.

Go to the Food Bank

If you work out, it's even more important to give potassium its proper respect.

You've probably heard that it's a good idea to eat a banana after a particularly strenuous workout. Why? Because potassium is essential for cell growth and for every pound of muscle you gain, your body needs more potassium.

It's also important because as an electrolyte, potassium is lost through sweat as well as urine. If you perspire, then you also have the potential to lose some potassium.

Increasing your potassium is as simple as peeling a banana or eating a nectarine. Experts agree that your body will respond better to potassium from food than to potassium taken in supplement form.

If you do decide to go with a supplement, check with your doctor first because low potassium levels can signal a variety of serious problems, including adrenal gland dysfunction, renal disorders, and intestinal dysfunction. Also, our bodies tolerate the various versions of potassium very differently. You can choose between potassium bicarbonate, potassium chloride, and potassium gluconate.

"It's often not necessary to go to such

Roll Away the Stone

Imagine a pea-size rock traveling ever so slowly through the small tube connecting your kidney to your bladder. Each time the pebble makes any progress, it gouges the tube (called the ureter), causing sharp, excruciating pain. Now picture the tiny rock pushing its way through your urethra (the tube that carries urine through the penis), all the while producing pain that can extend through the penis to the testicles and around to the lower back. This diabolical instrument of torture is the kidney stone.

Studies have shown that there is a way for men to cut in half their odds of developing this painful condition: Eat lots of fruits and vegetables rich in potassium.

"We've found potassium to be more protective than anything else," says Gary Curhan, M.D., chief of clinical nephrology at West Roxbury Veterans Affairs Medical Center in Massachusetts. So protective, in fact, that supplements including potassium are sometimes prescribed for chronic stone sufferers.

But you don't need supplements to get plenty of potassium. Eating five or more servings of fruits and vegetables a day will do nicely.

lengths as supplementation unless you are on certain medications that make you lose potassium or have a medical problem causing potassium deficiency," Dr. Ruml says. "Citrus fruits are better than pills. Drink a glass of orange juice or add lemons to your water." In fact, a glass of orange juice, grapefruit juice, carrot juice, or tomato juice will give you between 400 and 700 milligrams. And eating the five to nine servings of fruits and vegetables recommended daily in the Food Guide Pyramid should increase your potassium to about 3,500 milligrams daily.

Selenium

• *Where You Get It:* Lobster, clams, crabs, whole grains, Brazil nuts, oysters.

• *What It Does for You:* Selenium works with vitamin E as an antioxidant and binds with toxins in the body, somehow rendering them harmless.

• *What a Man Needs:* Daily Value of 70 micrograms.

• *Cautions:* Severe toxicity and deficiency are rare in the United States.

When a horse grazing in Kansas starts acting woozy and wobbly, his owner knows that he has eaten too much locoweed—a plant rich in selenium.

But while a horse in Kansas might be getting too much selenium, a horse in Florida might not get any at all—and both extremes are dangerous. The same is also true for people: Getting too much or too little selenium can be hazardous to your health.

"Selenium is an essential trace element that enters into an enzyme group that works primarily as an antioxidant defense system of the body," says Vladimir Badmaev, M.D., Ph.D., vice president of scientific and medical affairs for Sabinsa Corporation, a nutraceutical research company in Piscataway, New Jersey. Selenium deficiencies have been shown to compromise the body's ability to fight back against heart disease, cancer, and arthritis—in general, against chronic debilitating disorders.

Studies also have shown that highly infectious and fatal diseases, such as AIDS and the Ebola virus, thrive in areas where there are low levels of selenium in the soil and the population suffers from poor nutrition in general. According to one theory, viruses such as AIDS or Ebola use up the selenium reserves in the infected cell and then move on to another cell in "search" of selenium. This would explain the spreading of the infection throughout the body. Being on the top of the food chain, people from regions with low selenium levels in the soil will likely eat produce depleted of selenium and stand a lesser chance of defending themselves against the viral infections.

In general, the soil in states east of the Mississippi River and west of the Rockies is low in selenium.

Still, Dr. Badmaev believes that people, particularly in selenium-poor regions, should supplement at the recommended level of 50 to 200 micrograms of elemental selenium a day.

Other researchers agree with him. "There is evidence to suggest that supplementing up to 200 micrograms a day may prevent certain types of cancer," says Dr. Forrest Nielsen of the U.S. Department of Agriculture–Agricultural Research Service Grand Forks Human Nutrition Research Center. "However, supplementing in higher amounts could lead to problems." You should consult your doctor before taking more than 100 micrograms of selenium.

When researchers at the University of Arizona in Tucson gave 200-microgram selenium supplements to people with a history of skin cancer, they found that the supplements seemed to ward off lung, colorectal, and prostate cancers. But the supplements did not change the rates of skin cancer. All the people in the study, however, were from the eastern coastal plain of the United States, an area well-known for its lack of selenium-rich soil as well as its high rates of skin cancer.

If you do choose to supplement, Dr. Badmaev suggests combining a selenium supplement with vitamin E, beta-carotene, and vitamin A. Experimental evidence shows that persons with low levels of vitamin E, beta-carotene, and vitamin A—combined with low levels of selenium—are at higher risk of developing cancer. Selenium's antioxidant functions may enable it to terminate cancer cells, Dr. Badmaev says. So combining selenium with other antioxidants can improve the anti-cancer effect.

Sodium

• **Where You Get It:** Table salt, anchovies, bacon, bologna, pickles, Parmesan cheese.

• **What It Does for You:** Regulates and balances the amount of fluids outside the cells in your body. Aids in muscle contractions and nerve function.

• **What a Man Needs:** Daily Value of 2,400 milligrams.

• **Cautions:** Too much dietary salt over a long period of time can cause your body to lose excessive amounts of calcium. A high-salt diet can also lead to high blood pressure. Sometimes this doesn't show up until people reach their forties and fifties, and then to an even greater extent when they reach their sixties and seventies. Normally, sodium needs to be replaced in the body only if you have thrown up, had diarrhea, or were profusely sweating.

For years, sodium has been cast as the villain in the battle against high blood pressure. The reason is that scientists who conducted early studies on high blood pressure found that people who ate a lot of salt frequently had slightly higher blood pressure readings. The answer seemed obvious: Cut back on salt and you'd reduce your risk of high blood pressure. It didn't work out that way, though.

Further studies found that using less salt didn't guarantee a drop in blood pressure. In fact, one study in Germany found that a low-salt diet did not appear to lower blood pressure in about 80 percent of those involved. And another study at Albert Einstein College of Medicine and Cornell University Medical College, both in New York City, showed that men with high blood pressure who ate the least salt (about 5,000 milligrams) each day were four times more likely to have a heart attack—precisely the health consequence a low-salt diet was supposed to prevent—than those who ate more than twice as much salt every day.

These days researchers understand that high blood pressure (also known as hypertension) is more complicated than merely eating too much salt. They are more inclined to believe that low potassium, calcium, or magnesium levels as well as other lifestyle habits, such as exercise, alcohol use, and body weight, contribute more clearly to hypertension than sodium intake.

However, that doesn't change one very important fact: Excessive salt intake is potentially dangerous and, at the very least, seems pointless.

"I don't know what to make of the studies that find that salt isn't as important to hypertension, and I haven't changed my view on the subject," says Louis Tobian, M.D., head of the hypertension department at the University of Minnesota Hospital in Minneapolis.

"We have very clear numbers showing that Western societies that consume a lot of salt have higher blood pressure rates than those of primitive societies with little access to salt—but the case rates don't show up until people are in their forties or fifties," Dr. Tobian says.

However, that doesn't necessarily mean that your blood pressure will drop if you switch to a low-salt diet after years of eating a high-salt diet, Dr. Tobian cautions. Based on studies with rats, he believes that the reason blood pressure doesn't decrease is that the long-term, high-salt intake somehow produces irreversible changes in the brain, which helps regulate blood pressure.

Dr. Tobian believes that the discrepancy in study results may reflect the body's inability to adapt to a drop in sodium intakes. In other words, since it takes decades for high blood pressure to show up in the body, it would take just as long for sodium restriction to change hypertension rates. Even those researchers who found that excessive sodium restriction is unwarranted for the high blood pressure population concede that high sodium intake has little, if any, benefit.

So what should a person do? "There's no doubt that we get too much salt in our diets," according to Dr. Lisa Ruml of the University of Texas Southwestern Medical Center at Dallas.

"It's one of the first things we measure when we look at minerals in the body. It plays such a big role in calcium imbalances as well as other problems. And everyone should look at the total amount they eat every day to see if they can cut back," Dr. Ruml adds.

That's because aside from its association with high blood pressure, too much dietary sodium can threaten your body's store of calcium. And that can lead to osteoporosis later in life.

Both potassium and calcium work to lower blood pressure, but when too much sodium is in the blood, it forces the levels of potassium and calcium down.

It Ain't Easy

Sodium is one-half of table salt, that ubiquitous taste enhancer flavoring everything from sushi to American cheese. It is also a mineral within our bodies, an electrolyte to be exact, which means that it dissolves in liquid. Half the sodium in your body is within your blood vessels and in fluids surrounding your cells, another 40 percent is on the surface of your bones, and the remaining 10 percent is in your cells.

Although our taste for excess salt seems

Packaged Goods

If you want to know at a glance how much sodium a product contains, here's what the terms on the front of the package mean.

Sodium-free: **less than 5 milligrams per serving**

Very low sodium: **no more than 35 milligrams per serving**

Low-sodium: **fewer than 140 milligrams per serving**

Less sodium: **25 percent less per serving than similar food**

Light: **50 percent or less per serving than the regular product**

---

to be acquired, human beings appear to crave a certain level of sodium. Most Americans get about 3,000 to 6,000 milligrams each day, well above the Daily Value of 2,400 milligrams. "Ideally, you'd like to keep your intake to the Daily Value, which means about a half-inch of salt from a diner-style saltshaker," Dr. Ruml says. This amount includes the salt that's already in the foods you eat. Most people eat about an inch of salt a day.

But the problem isn't caused by the salt you shake on your food; it's the salt stirred in much earlier that causes the problem. Canned chicken noodle soup? Around 1,000 milligrams a serving. Lunchmeat? About 350 milligrams a slice. You get the picture.

"It's difficult to control your salt consumption if you eat out a lot," adds Dr. Ruml. "Sodium is a great preservative. Restaurants and food manufacturers tend to use a lot of it.

"Look at the label and count up how much you're eating in a day," advises Dr. Ruml. "Don't worry about each serving at first. Instead, focus on your total. Aim to keep the amount in the 2- to 3-gram range, rather than having it push up to 5 grams or more."

Zinc

• **Where You Get It:** Meats, poultry, eggs, dairy products, oysters, spices.

• **What It Does for You:** Essential for normal growth, development, and immunity. Helps maintain skin, hair, and bones. Keeps the reproductive organs functioning and helps in the perception of taste and the ability to see at night.

• **What a Man Needs:** Daily Value of 15 milligrams.

• **Cautions:** Ingesting 2 grams or more of zinc can make you sick to your stomach. Long-term, elevated levels of zinc can cause anemia, lower your immunity, and interfere with your body's ability to absorb two other essential minerals—copper and iron.

So, was lunch tasty today? Did you really enjoy the steak you had for dinner last night? Thank zinc. This trace mineral has a lot to do with your ability to taste. In fact, zinc plays a large role in anything that exists on the surface area of the body, such as skin, hair, mucous membranes, and taste buds.

You probably know more about zinc's reputation as an aphrodisiac. Supposedly, zinc will improve a man's sex life by increasing his potency.

"Rats that have been raised on virtually no zinc at all have a problem with sperm production," says Dr. Janet Hunt of the U.S. Department of Agriculture–Agricultural Research Service Grand Forks Human Nutrition Research Center. "But in humans there's only a difference in seed speed, as we call it, if we've completely depleted the body of zinc. That would rarely happen in an American man eating a typical American diet."

What happens if you suddenly take zinc out of a normal diet? One study at Wayne State University in Detroit, with 40 men ages 20 to 80, showed that when men's daily intake of zinc was cut back, the amount of testosterone they produced also dropped substantially. Testosterone is the most important male sex hormone, responsible for development of the male reproductive organs, including the prostate. It also helps maintain muscle strength and the growth of bone and muscle.

While depletion of zinc is rare, a slight zinc deficiency is common for older men, people on diets, vegetarians, and people who drink a lot of alcohol, exercise a lot, or who are under a lot of stress. That's because zinc is easily lost through urine and sweat. Symptoms of a zinc shortage include white spots in the fingernails, dull-colored hair, stunted growth, skin changes, delayed wound healing, and small sex glands in young boys.

"Overt zinc deficiency is quite dramatic," Dr. Hunt says. "There is a reduction in growth in children, failure to repair tissues, and dermatitis."

Since there are no stores of zinc in the body, getting the right amount from your diet and possibly supplementation is very important. "Zinc helps keep the skin healthy and intact. If you get enough zinc, blood will flow to your skin more easily," says Dr. Lisa Ruml of the University of Texas Southwestern Medical Center at Dallas. "People prone to canker sores may benefit from taking zinc, too."

A number of things can inhibit zinc absorption, including too much calcium and copper as well as phytic acid and fiber in food. Phytic acid is a phosphorous compound that can bind to zinc and carry it out of the body. It's found in whole grains but not in meats, which is one reason why animal products are better sources of zinc than plant foods.

"You should still eat whole grains because the zinc in grains can add to the zinc found in meats," Dr. Hunt says. "Vegetarians are at risk because their only source of zinc is grains." Most foods have the correct ratio of zinc and copper, which will prevent the minerals from counteracting one another. But not all supplements include both. This can be a problem, Dr. Hunt warns.

While whole-wheat bread will have some zinc, the mineral is removed from processed flour and is not replaced in cereal or bread.

Can Zinc Zap the Common Cold?

Maybe vitamin C has a better press agent. When it comes to the common cold, vitamin C gets all the accolades. But there is increasing evidence that zinc gluconate may have true star potential.

"We've known since 1984 that zinc gluconate could soothe sore throats and decrease the severity of colds," says John C. Godfrey, Ph.D., president of Godfrey Science and Design in Huntingdon Valley, Pennsylvania. "The problem was that the taste was repulsive."

So, Dr. John C. Godfrey and his wife, Nancy J. Godfrey, Ph.D., did what any good scientists or inventors would do. They turned to the recipes of candy-makers. But none of the ideas involving sugar or ascorbic acid panned out.

"I had to find a way to fix the flavor and not let the zinc's effectiveness suffer," says Dr. John C. Godfrey. "There's a small amino acid called glycine that has a very pleasant taste. It's what makes meat, particularly lamb, taste good." Voilà! Dr. Godfrey had his patent, and Cold-Eezer Plus was born.

Make no mistake, Cold-Eezer Plus—which debuted on the market in the winter of 1994–1995 and has since been revised as Cold-Eeze—still has a strong taste. But let it dissolve in your mouth and your throat will feel better. If you swallow the tablets, there is no effect.

"You want to have lots of zinc ions in

> ## Put Zinc on Your Nose
>
> Not only does zinc work in your nose and throat but also it works on your skin to prevent sunburn. Zinc oxide, that white stuff you see on the face of lifeguards, won't let the sun's dangerous ultraviolet rays permeate the skin.
>
> "Zinc oxide is insoluble," says Dr. Nancy J. Godfrey of Godfrey Science and Design. That means that it won't dissolve in water—a helpful characteristic, indeed, when you're at the ocean.

---

the mouth and nose," says Sabrina Novick, Ph.D., assistant professor of chemistry at Hofstra University in Hempstead, New York.

Why? Dr. Novick explains it this way: When it comes to your cold's progression, the rhinovirus associated with the common cold contains the lock and your cells have the key. They attract each other. The positively charged zinc ion temporarily blocks the key from entering the lock. But it is only temporary. That's why you need to take another lozenge every 2 to 4 hours. "It's not curing the cold. It's stopping the progression," Dr. Novick says.

The bottom line, according to Dr. John C. Godfrey, is that the zinc lozenges—taken correctly—can cut the duration of your cold in half. However, you have to start taking the lozenges as soon as you feel a little tickle in your throat to get the full effect.

Taking one Cold-Eeze every 3 to 4 hours, as recommended by the manufacturer, will give you more than the Daily Value for zinc over the course of a day. This is harmless for the few days it takes to treat a cold, says Dr. John C. Godfrey. Safety of the new "second generation" lozenges is increased by the addition of a trace of copper, just sufficient enough to reverse any possible zinc interference if lozenges are used for more than a few days. These lozenges are only meant to be taken for a short period of time, so be sure not to exceed the manufacturer's directions.

The Best of the Rest

Copper

• **Where You Get It:** Black pepper, blackstrap molasses, Brazil nuts, cocoa.

• **What It Does for You:** Helps prevent anemia by assisting the body to release and absorb iron. Contributes to the release of energy, the synthesis of red blood cells (hemoglobin) and the proteins collagen and elastin, the neurotransmitter noradrenaline, and the pigment in your hair.

• **What a Man Needs:** Daily Value of 2 milligrams.

• **Cautions:** Numerous other minerals, including calcium, iron, lead, and zinc, reduce the utilization of copper. Toxicity occurs when water or other beverages have been stored in copper containers.

When it comes to building a strong body, copper is like pennies from heaven. Too bad most of us act as if the precious mineral was only worth one red cent.

"Copper is an element that doesn't receive as much attention as it deserves because we haven't looked at it in the right way," says Dr. Forrest Nielsen of the U.S. Department of Agriculture–Agricultural Research Service Grand Forks Human Nutrition Research Center. "There's no good way to indicate if a person is deficient. I believe that many people are consuming less than 1 milligram a day and that low consumption has a detrimental effect on cardiovascular and bone health."

Copper plays a role in the body's formation of strong, flexible connective tissue; in the production of neurochemicals in the brain; and in the functioning of muscles, nerves, and the immune system. Your body stores most of its copper in your bloodstream. However, other minerals—most notably zinc—can interfere with your body's ability to absorb copper.

"The healthy ratio for zinc to copper is in the range of 8 to 12 parts of zinc to 1 part of copper," says Alexander Schauss, Ph.D., director of the life sciences division of the American Institute for Biosocial Research in Tacoma, Washington, and author of *Minerals, Trace Elements, and Human Health*. "Other things can also lead to an imbalance of copper in your body, including smoking cigarettes, having a lot of stress, and drinking tea." Since tea is a diuretic, it drains the body of trace elements, Dr. Schauss says.

Research has shown that too little copper leads to anemia, a disease involving decreased levels of hemoglobin in red blood cells, and also tiny or a reduced number of red blood cells. Early symptoms include fatigue. Dr. Schauss says that excesses of copper, usually as a result of high levels in water, contribute to incidences of hyperactivity in children. In adults, getting too much copper (more than 3 milligrams a day) can cause vomiting.

Fluoride

• **Where You Get It:** Fluoridated water and toothpaste, seaweed, marine fish with bones, tea.

• **What It Does for You:** Prevents cavities and helps make bone tissue stronger.

• **What a Man Needs:** Estimated Safe and Adequate Daily Dietary Intake of 1.5 to 4 milligrams.

• *Cautions:* Excess fluoride causes the enamel of developing teeth to become chalky and mottled-looking. Deficiency of fluoride results in excess dental cavities in people of all ages and possibly more osteoporosis in older folks.

Unless you're like Jack Nicholson's pain-loving freak in the original film version of *The Little Shop of Horrors*, you'd probably be perfectly content to live the rest of your days without ever hearing the sound of a dentist's drill again. If that's the case, don't make the mistake of thinking that fluoride was something you only needed while sprouting your permanent teeth way back when. It turns out that fluoride is as important to men of 40 as it is to a boy of 4.

"Sometimes men begin to get more cavities around the age of 40," says Israel Kleinberg, D.D.S., Ph.D., professor and chairman of the department of oral biology and pathology at the School of Dental Medicine at the State University of New York at Stony Brook. "It's usually because either stress or a medication they're taking has caused them to have a drier mouth with less saliva."

Your teeth are more susceptible to the acids in food and drink without enough saliva swishing around, so there is a danger of mineral loss. The fluoride in toothpaste and drinking water can help.

"Keep using fluoridated toothpaste, even if you think you're past the years of getting cavities," Dr. Kleinberg says. "Fluoride can always help."

There is an abundance of evidence supporting fluoride's role in warding off cavities. Ideally, between your water supply, fluoride toothpaste, and other tooth products with fluoride, such as mouthwash, adults should try to get between 1.5 and 4 milligrams of fluoride a day. Kids four years old and up, however, should get no more than 2.5 milligrams a day because more can damage teeth, according to the Estimated Safe and Adequate Daily Dietary Intakes of the National Research Council.

"Fluorosis, a mottling pattern on the teeth, only effects tooth enamel during its formation," Dr. Kleinberg says. "Between fluoridated water, juices made with fluoridated water, and toothpaste, children can get too much."

Aside from your teeth, fluoride has been shown to aid in your body's drive to maintain its calcium stores in your bones. While the fluoride in your toothpaste can't help, there will soon be tablets of slow-release sodium fluoride that have proven effective.

One study showed that people who took the slow-release fluoride in conjunction with calcium citrate supplements decreased the rate of spinal fractures in women who were prone to them because of low-density bone levels. The use of slow-release fluoride as a drug to help fight osteoporosis is still being examined. What does that mean? Men—who develop osteoporosis later in life than women—may one day find themselves considering this kind of supplementation.

Iodine

• *Where You Get It:* Iodized salt, lobster, shrimp, breads, milk.

• *What It Does for You:* Iodine has only one function: to make the hormones secreted by the thyroid gland.

• *What a Man Needs:* Daily Value of 150 micrograms.

• *Cautions:* Oddly enough, too much and too little can lead to an enlargement of the thyroid gland, known as goiter.

The thyroid gland uses iodine to produce thyroxine, a key hormone that helps regulate energy production, body temperature, breathing, muscle tone, and the manufacture and breakdown of tissues. Iodine deficiency and excess usually result in goiter, an enlargement of the thyroid gland that is visible as swelling on the front of the neck.

With iodine-fortified salt, most—but not all—of us easily get more than the Daily Value of 150 micrograms.

"There are a few areas in this country that still have cases of goiter," says Dr. Schauss. "Mostly in mountainous regions, such as the Appalachians." Studies have shown that microorganisms can cause goiter, rather than iodine deficiency itself. However, iodine deficiency in the soil and water is the major cause of goiter. It may be an organism, similar to ones such as *Salmonella* or *Escherichia coli*, he says.

The most interesting thing about iodine, according to Dr. Schauss, is its role in brain function. "We've found that children who are exposed to radiation, or iodine 131 (I_{131}), have more trouble in school," he says. In fact, when the Soviet Union's nuclear power plant at Chernobyl exploded, the Polish government handed out iodine tablets to everyone in Poland within 3 to 4 days.

Other governments such as Sweden and Italy urged their citizens to consume kelp or iodine supplements to protect their thyroid from exposure to I_{131}. Kelp contains iodine 192, the stable form of iodine we find in our salt.

Manganese

• *Where You Get It:* Brown rice, spices, nuts, whole grains, beans, blueberries.

• *What It Does for You:* Helps form bones and stimulates growth of connective tissue. Assists in the synthesis of fatty acids, cholesterol, and the activation of various enzymes. Thought to have some role in brain function.

• *What a Man Needs:* Daily Value of 2 milligrams.

• *Cautions:* The body absorbs only about 45 percent of consumed manganese from the average diet.

Sometimes good things do come in small packages. Take manganese, a mineral found in humans, animals, plants—and even gingerbread men. Eat a few cookies and you will get a good dose of this humble, yet powerful, element.

Manganese—derived from the Greek word for magic—itself isn't an ingredient of gingerbread cookies. But cloves and ginger are, and they feature whopping doses of manganese. Aside from its role in holiday baking, manganese also is used as an alloy in the production of steel to give it toughness. Go figure.

This is one of those minerals where you're far more likely to get too much than too little. There's only been one documented case of manganese deficiency, but there have been lots of toxicity reports.

That's because miners and other people who work around minerals have been known to inhale the stuff. It can be poisonous in this form. However, toxicity from ingestion is rare but has been caused by contaminated drinking water or from taking high doses of a dietary supplement.

This also is one of those minerals where you probably should get more than the Daily Value, which is just 2 milligrams, says Dr. Schauss. However, if you plan to take more than 10 milligrams a day, consult with your doctor first.

Although manganese has not been studied very often, and rarely with humans, it has been shown to play a role in metabolism, glucose tolerance, insulin response, and brain function. Manganese is found in the mitochondria, our energy cells. And without manganese, the energy might remain stuck.

"Animals with high levels of manganese show higher levels of antisocial behavior," says Dr. Schauss. "Unfortunately, we're more than a decade away from understanding the extent of this relationship."

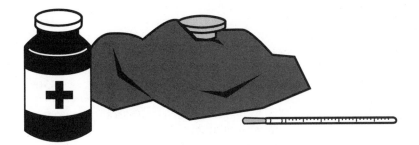

Part Four

Healing with Vitamins

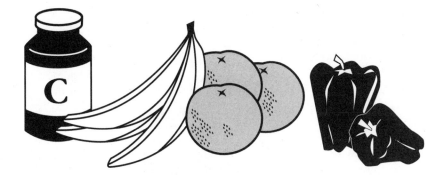

Allergies

Taming the Savage Sneeze

Faster than a speeding bullet. More powerful than a locomotive. Able to make its victims itch, wheeze, sneeze, weep, cough, and ache in a single attack. Is it the flu? Is it food poisoning? No, it's your pesky allergies bringing you to your knees again.

Allergies can lay waste a mere mortal the way kryptonite fells Superman. The list of potential allergens—substances that people can be allergic to—is quite long: from pollen, cat dander, and dust mites to such seemingly harmless substances as strawberries, shaving cream, and fabrics. The symptoms are just as versatile, affecting the nose, eyes, throat, lungs, stomach, skin, or nervous system, or even causing fatigue or depression—all of which can hit you in varying strengths.

You might not think of yourself as oversensitive, but sometimes the immune system is. Allergy symptoms occur when your body's immune system overreacts to substances you're exposed to. Histamine and leukotrienes, powerful defensive chemicals that your immune system releases, can cause many of the common allergy symptoms, including runny nose and nasal congestion. Mast cells—found in tissues such as skin, lungs, throat, stomach, and intestines—release histamine. And cells called basophils, which hang out in your blood vessels, release leukotrienes when they are exposed to an allergen.

Of course, the best way to put an end to your allergy troubles is to avoid the allergens that affect you in the first place and to take any allergy medicine that your doctor prescribes. But some nutrients may be able to prevent some of your misery,

too, provided they are taken before an allergy attack. Here's what the experts say about the most promising ones.

Vitamin C: The Bodyguard

Vitamin C's effect on allergic reactions has been heavily studied. High levels of vitamin C help reduce histamine release from mast cells and also make histamine break down faster once it is released. And when you're low on vitamin C, researchers discovered, your blood levels of histamine rise. But investigators are now seeing a broader picture of just how vitamin C may affect the allergic-reaction process, and there's evidence that it doesn't work alone.

Enter bioflavonoids. Plant foods contain more than 4,000 of these unique natural chemicals, and researchers have been investigating their role in allergy prevention for decades. "Vitamin C works as an antioxidant that protects the bioflavonoids, which look to be what's really reducing the allergy symptoms," says Jeremy E. Kaslow, M.D., assistant clinical professor of medicine at the University of California, Irvine, and an allergy specialist in Garden Grove, California.

It's too early for scientists to make specific recommendations about the kinds or exact amount of bioflavonoids that people with allergies should be taking, says Elliott Middleton Jr., M.D., professor emeritus of medicine at the State University of New York at Buffalo School of Medicine and Biomedical Sciences and founder of the Chebeague Island Institute of Natural Product Research in Maine. But it's still a good idea to regularly consume foods that contain bioflavonoids. They aren't hard to come by if you are eating right to begin with, says Dr. Middleton.

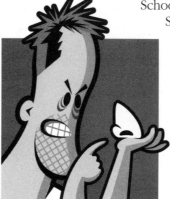

"Foods with vitamin C have bioflavonoids by default, so diet can be a means of getting enough of both nutrients," Dr. Kaslow says. Getting the recommended five to nine servings of fruits and vegetables should make it easy to reach the Daily Value for vitamin C (60 milligrams) and provide a healthy dose of bioflavonoids at the same time. Some doctors suggest that getting 1,000 to 2,000 milligrams of vitamin C a day is beneficial to ward off some allergy symptoms.

Dr. Kaslow recommends that if you are taking a supplement with vitamin C for allergy relief, make sure that the product label also says that it contains bioflavonoids.

Mighty Magnesium

Magnesium helps to relieve bronchospasm, or constricted airways, in the lungs. It has been used intravenously to help relieve the symptoms of life-threatening, drug-resistant asthma attacks. Now it seems that this mineral may be valuable in keeping histamines in check.

"The flow of calcium into and out of a cell helps regulate some cell function. Magnesium deficiency may change the permeability of mast cell membranes, allowing calcium to enter cells more easily," says Kay Franz, Ph.D., associate professor of nutrition at Brigham Young University in Provo, Utah, and one of the study's authors. "When that happens, histamine is released."

Regardless of whether you suffer from allergies, experts recommend that you get your Daily Value of 400 milligrams of magnesium. That's because magnesium is an important player in many of the body's functions. Foods like nuts, beans, whole grains, bananas, and green vegetables will help. Don't go overboard with magnesium, though, unless you're ready to put in a lot of extra hours sitting on the toilet. It is, after all, what gives milk of magnesia its laxative powers.

If you have kidney problems and are considering taking a magnesium supplement, check with your doctor first. Most people with kidney disease have a decreased ability to clear waste products from the blood. Excess magnesium in the diet or from supplements would not be easily excreted and could build up in the blood and tissues to potentially toxic levels.

Remember the Membrane

Now here's a sticky subject. The mucous lining is the body's internal skin. It is a layer of cells containing infection-fighting biochemicals that secrete mucus, that slimy substance revered by prepubescent boys. Mucus has an important function: It shields cells from direct contact with pollen and other allergens.

"Having an unhealthy mucous lining will promote allergies," says Dr. Kaslow. So make sure that you're effectively sliming those attacking allergens by consuming adequate amounts of vitamin A (or its precursor, beta-carotene), selenium, iodine, and zinc. "Those are the ones that we focus on when there is a problem with mucus, but you still need to have good supplies of all nutrients to have a consistently healthy mucous lining," explains Dr. Kaslow.

Antioxidants: Can They Help?

An allergic reaction causes the generation of unstable molecules called free radicals, which injure your body's healthy molecules by stealing electrons to balance themselves. In the process free radicals injure mast cells and may make them even more twitchy and prone to histamine release, says Dr. Middleton. Vitamins C and E, beta-carotene, selenium, and other antioxidants all help to neutralize free radicals by offering their own electrons, thus protecting healthy molecules from harm.

It is still unknown how much of which antioxidants is needed to have an effect on allergic reactions, so Dr. Middleton suggests that people make sure that they are eating lots of fresh fruits and vegetables that are rich in antioxidants. "There may be undiscovered nutrients at work alone or in tandem with known antioxidants in whole foods," he explains.

Arthritis

Vitamins May Ease Pain

Arthritis affects nearly 40 million Americans, one-third of whom are men. Of the more than 100 types of arthritis, the two most prevalent kinds that show up in men are rheumatoid arthritis and osteoarthritis. Rheumatoid arthritis is an autoimmune disease where the lining of the joints becomes inflamed. It can affect other internal organs as well and can move from one area of the body to another over time. Osteoarthritis, also called degenerative joint disease, causes the breakdown of the cartilage in a particular joint that results in pain and stiffness.

Stopping Progress

Treating the effects of arthritis requires a combination of therapies, including medications, heat, exercise, and in some cases, surgery. Although no nutritional measures can replace these treatments, there is some promising news from experts on vitamins and minerals that may ease some of your arthritis pain. Here's what you need to know.

Vitamin C

A group of researchers observed the eating habits of 640 people with and without osteoarthritis of the knee over the course of eight years. They found that those who consumed the most vitamin C had three times less disease progression than people eating the least of the vitamin. "Vitamin C helps body tissues repair themselves, which may explain why people who ate more of this nutrient had less progression of the disease," says study leader Tim McAlindon, M.D., assistant professor of medicine at Boston

University School of Medicine and the Boston University Arthritis Center.

"From our study, 120 milligrams—or twice the current Daily Value—seems to be enough vitamin C to bring you up to levels where the most osteoarthritis benefits were reported," says Dr. McAlindon. That's about the equivalent of two oranges. It's still too early to recommend large intakes of vitamin C to all osteoarthritis sufferers, however.

"We also saw some effect from two other antioxidants we looked at, vitamin E and beta-carotene, although vitamin C was the strongest and most consistent," Dr. McAlindon says. Further studies would be necessary, however, before any recommendations could be made for these nutrients.

Vitamin D

Dr. McAlindon also published a similar study that looked at the relationship between vitamin D consumption and the progression of osteoarthritis in the knee. When high dietary intakes of vitamin D were reported among the 556 participants in the eight-year study, there was a fourfold reduction in the progression of the disease. When blood serum levels of the vitamin were measured, those with high levels of vitamin D were 2½ times less likely to suffer from osteoarthritis progression.

Vitamin D is synthesized through your skin by the action of ultraviolet light that is present in sunlight and is also found in herring, salmon, sardines, and fortified milks and cereals. Dr. McAlindon says that it's too early to start recommending large doses of this potentially toxic vitamin. He doesn't see any harm, however, in getting the Daily Value for vitamin D (400 international units).

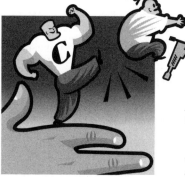

Vitamin B$_{12}$ and Folic Acid

In a study of 26 patients with osteoarthritis, sufferers tried a two-month regimen each of folic acid supplements; vitamin B$_{12}$ and folic acid supplements; and placebos. Only when the combination pill was taken did researchers see greatly improved hand grip and strength in patients. All the participants were off anti-arthritis medications for 10 days prior to the double-blind trials (that means that the researcher and the participants had no idea who got which pills until the study was over).

"The B$_{12}$/folic acid combination was just as good from a pain stand-point as taking nonsteroidal anti-inflammatory drugs and didn't have the side effects associated with those medications," says Margaret Flynn, R.D., Ph.D., professor of family and community medicine at the University of Missouri–Columbia School of Medicine in Columbia, and lead investigator of the study.

Vitamin B$_{12}$ helps induce new bone formation that can help relieve the immobility and pain that osteoarthritis causes, but it can only function in this capacity with the help of folate (the natural form of folic acid found in food). While more studies are needed before recommendations can be set, Dr. Flynn says that some physicians are already prescribing dosages like the ones given in her study: 6,400 micrograms (6.4 milligrams) of folic acid and 20 micrograms of vitamin B$_{12}$. "That's a good, safe level," she says.

Check with your doctor before taking more than the Daily Value of B$_{12}$ (6 micrograms), especially if you have folate deficiency, iron deficiency, or any kind of infection. Doses of more than the Daily Value for folate (400 micrograms) can mask the symptoms of pernicious anemia, a vitamin B$_{12}$ deficiency, so check with your doctor before supplementing with folic acid.

Something Fishy

Perhaps the most compelling nutritional research regarding arthritis has come in the area of omega-3 fatty acids, which are compounds in fish oils that ease rheumatoid arthritis.

More than 15 well-designed scientific studies worldwide have documented the significant beneficial results from taking fish oils for rheumatoid arthritis. Researchers from Albany Medical College in Albany, New York, found that patients who took fish-oil capsules as well as standard arthritis medication had significantly fewer tender joints and less morning stiffness than patients taking corn-oil capsules.

"There is very good, sound scientific evidence and rationale behind the improvements that we see," says Joel Kremer, M.D., professor of medicine and head of the division of rheumatology at Albany Medical College. "But it takes three to five months before you can really start to see benefits, and you have to take a lot."

To get results over this period of time, you'll need to take 3 to 5 grams of omega-3 fatty acids, which for most supplements means 8 to 14 capsules a day. Just remember: It's only effective if you continue to take your current arthritis medications, Dr. Kremer says.

Look for fish-oil capsules that list the omega-3 fatty acids EPA (eicosapentaenoic acid) and DHA (docosahexaenoic acid) on the label. You'll also need to take vitamin E with any supplements of fish oils, so make sure that's on the label as well. Vitamin E, an antioxidant, protects the omega-3 fatty acids from being destroyed by oxidation. Make sure to talk to your doctor before starting to take large doses of any nutritional supplement.

Cancer

Tilting the Odds in Your Favor

For years, many men viewed cancer as a cosmic game of Russian roulette. If the bullet had your name on it, there was nothing you could do about it. But over the years, research has shown that there is something you can do about it. Something that might boost the odds by nearly 35 percent in your favor. And it's something that you do every single day: eating.

Just about everything you put in your mouth can play a role, positive or negative, when it comes to cancer. If you're still playing Russian roulette, think of it this way: You can either load extra bullets into the chambers or take precautions to keep the number of loaded chambers to a minimum. The choice is yours.

Food for Thought

Understand first that there is no magic pill that will protect you against cancer. Supplementing smartly for certain key nutrients appears to help, but only if you're eating a well-balanced, healthy diet that is low in fat and high in fiber and includes plenty of fruits and vegetables.

"I think that there is probably a complex mixture of ingredients in foods that help to thwart or reduce the risk of cancer. There's interest in many compounds in plant foods that might be interacting to help prevent cancer," says Allen Vegotsky, Ph.D., scientific program director in the American Cancer Society's research department in Atlanta. For these reasons, organizations looking to help prevent cancer recommend the following National Cancer Institute guidelines.

- Reduce fat intake to 30 percent of calories or less.
- Increase fiber to 20 to 30 grams per day, with an upper limit of 35 grams.
- Include a variety of fruits and vegetables in your daily diet.
- Avoid obesity.
- Consume alcoholic beverages in moderation, if at all.
- Minimize consumption of salt-cured, salt-pickled, and smoked foods.

While smoking is not a nutritional consideration, it is a prominent risk factor for cancer, Dr. Vegotsky says. "In my opinion, quitting smoking is as important as diet and exercise and is much more important than taking a vitamin supplement," he says.

But provided that you're nicotine-free, supplements can play an important role. One study involving almost 30,000 men and women in China found that death rates from cancer dropped by 13 percent among those taking supplements of beta-carotene, vitamin E, and selenium. Death rates specifically from stomach cancer and lung cancer went down 21 percent and 45 percent, respectively. Additional studies have supported these findings as well as a connection between vitamin C and reduced risk of various types of cancer. In addition, antioxidants play a crucial role in ensuring that our immune systems are at optimal strength to attack tumor cells that may begin to develop in our bodies, says James Anderson, M.D., professor of medicine and clinical nutrition at the University of Kentucky in Lexington and author of Dr. Anderson's Antioxidant Antiaging Health Program.

There are more than 100 different kinds of cancers, with varying treatments and risk factors. Modern science understands cancer to be a multistage process. There's an initiation stage, where some compound or physical force alters the genetic material in our bodies. Next is the promotion stage, in which a series of mutations and changes occur in a cell before it becomes cancerous. In the final phase, known as progression, pre-cancerous cells develop into cancerous ones, which lead to out-of-control growth and tumor development.

Supplementing Smartly

Scientists have long been interested in tapping into the powers of nutrients to prevent and combat cancer in its many stages and forms. Here are the most promising areas they've identified.

Vitamin C

Diets high in vitamin C–rich fruits and vegetables are associated with a lower risk of several forms of cancer, according to an examination of published vitamin C and vitamin E studies on cancer. Researchers found that these diets also are associated with at least a 40 percent lower risk for cancers of the gastrointestinal tract and lungs, specifically. Vitamin C may also help reduce the risk of stomach, mouth, and pancreas cancers, Dr. Anderson says. Besides having its own cancer-fighting properties, vitamin C may work to restore vitamin E—another anti-cancer antioxidant—after it has been damaged by free radicals, says Dr. Anderson.

The current Daily Value for vitamin C is 60 milligrams. "I think that vitamin C is where we will see the next major breakthrough in terms of upward movement of the recommendations," Dr. Anderson says. Until then, besides taking a multivitamin/mineral supplement, Dr. Anderson advises taking 250 milligrams of vitamin C twice a day for general cancer protection. If you have a strong family history of cancer or have been diagnosed with

Calcium and Colon Cancer

Getting enough calcium may do more than just help keep your bones strong. It may also help keep your colon clear of cancer. Population studies suggest that people who get lots of calcium-rich foods in their diets are less likely than normal to develop colon cancer.

Calcium may thwart colon cancer by binding with cancer-promoting fats and bile acids, the digestive fluid secreted by the liver, says Bernard Levin, M.D., professor of medicine and vice president for cancer prevention at the University of Texas M. D. Anderson Cancer Center in Houston. This neutralizes their toxic effects and causes them to be excreted without harming intestinal cells, he says.

"These effects seem to be strongest in people at highest risk for colon cancer, those eating high-fat diets," Dr. Levin says. People who eat low-fat diets, whose risk may already be low, don't benefit as much from additional calcium.

Several studies of people at high risk for colon cancer—such as those with a prior history of polyps, benign growths that can lead to cancer—also suggest that calcium may help reduce the possibility of abnormal growth in the cells lining the colon.

Don't count on miracles, however, Dr. Levin warns. "The effects are fairly modest and occur only at amounts well above normal intake," he says. Most studies used 1,250 milligrams a day, while the average daily intake of calcium is less than 800 milligrams. The Daily Value for calcium is 1,000 milligrams.

some type of the disease, boost your vitamin C supplementation up to 500 milligrams twice a day, Dr. Anderson says. Just be aware that large doses of vitamin C can cause diarrhea.

Vitamin E

Animal studies have consistently shown that vitamin E can help protect cells from damage that can lead to cancer. Human studies have had mixed results in the past, but emerging long-term trials are promising. This nutrient may help reduce the risk of stomach cancer and lung cancer, and because it is soluble in fats, vitamin E can protect lipid membranes from oxidation damage, Dr. Anderson says.

In addition to taking a multivitamin/mineral supplement, Dr. Anderson advises taking 400 international units (IU) of vitamin E a day for general cancer protection. But if you have a strong family history of cancer, or have already been diagnosed with some type of the disease, he recommends taking up to 800 IU of vitamin E daily.

However, doses over 600 IU should only be taken under a doctor's supervision. If you are taking anticoagulant drugs, consult your doctor before taking supplements of vitamin E over 400 IU.

Beta-Carotene

Beta-carotene appears to protect parts of the body by limiting the promotion phase of cancer development. It appears to be particularly effective in protecting against cancers of the lung and oral cavity, Dr. Anderson says. And because it is a fat-soluble antioxidant, beta-carotene protects lipid membranes from oxidative damage, he says.

Beta-carotene received some very bad press when three studies (one Finnish; one called the Carotene and Retinol Efficacy Trial, or CARET; and one called the Physicians Health Study) reported that men receiving beta-carotene actually developed cancer at a greater, or no-better, rate than men getting placebos.

Folic Acid Reduces Risk

Not all nutrients linked to cancer risk reduction are antioxidants. Just look at folic acid. Found in many vegetables, beans, fruits, whole grains, and fortified breakfast cereals, folic acid—known as folate when found naturally in foods—may reduce the risk of some cancers.

Researchers from Harvard Medical School found that high folic acid levels in the diet were associated with reduced risk of precancerous colorectal polyps, compared to diets getting low levels of the nutrient. Other studies have drawn similar conclusions. Researchers at the University of Alabama found that smokers treated with 10 milligrams (10,000 micrograms) of folic acid and 500 micrograms of vitamin B_{12} each day had significantly fewer precancerous cells than an untreated group. (Vitamin B_{12} was added because smokers tend to be deficient in B_{12} and because folic acid needs B_{12} to be active.)

Another study, conducted by Japanese doctors, found that folic acid and vitamin B_{12} provide impressive protection. Smokers who took 10 to 20 milligrams (10,000 to 20,000 micrograms) of folic acid and 750 micrograms of B_{12} daily had significant reductions in the number of potentially precancerous cells found in abnormal spots in the passage-

Health groups and the media were quick to bash beta-carotene supplements, says Dr. Anderson. But perhaps they were too fast to judge. In two of the studies, a significant increase in risk was seen in men who were smokers, not men who were nonsmokers (one study actually saw a reduction in risk in former smokers who took beta-carotene supplements). Extremely high dosages of beta-carotene, or perhaps the method of administering the supplements, may also have contributed to the troubling findings. In any event, Dr. Anderson, along with other specialists in the antioxidant

ways of their lungs. The spots were checked with a lung-scanning scope several times over the course of one year. Seventy percent of initially abnormal spots were reclassified as normal by the end of the year, and not one lesion had gotten worse. In contrast, a control group that took no supplements fared this way: 77 percent of their spots remained the same, 5 percent got worse, and 18 percent got better.

"Folic acid deficiency may not be a true cancer-causing agent, but I think it may set cells up for the development of cancer," says Warren Heston, Ph.D., director of the George M. O'Brien Urology Center at Memorial Sloan-Kettering Cancer Center in New York City.

While he doesn't think men should take megadoses, Dr. Heston thinks that making sure you get at least the current Daily Value of folic acid (400 micrograms) each day is important. Going as high as 800 micrograms may even be a good idea for people with a family history of cancer, but check with your doctor because folic acid intake above 400 micrograms may mask signs of a B_{12} deficiency. Very large doses of folic acid have been linked to enhanced tumor growth, however, says Dr. Heston, so don't assume that more is better.

increasing your beta-carotene supplementation to 20,000 IU daily. Produce with a deep yellow or deep orange flesh such as sweet potatoes, carrots, and cantaloupe, and dark green, leafy vegetables such as spinach tend to be higher in the nutrient. Since many other cancer-fighting carotenoids exist in these types of plant foods, eating a wide variety each day is important.

Selenium

Animal studies have suggested that selenium, an antioxidant mineral found in grain products, protects against cancer. In a study led by Larry Clark, Ph.D., of the Arizona Cancer Center in Tucson, 1,312 people with a history of skin cancer were given either 200 micrograms of high-selenium yeast (a supplement) or a placebo over the course of 10 years. Although there did not appear to be any impact on skin cancer, the total cancer risk in the selenium group was almost 37 percent less than the group that got the fake pills. The selenium group also had a 50 percent reduction in cancer mortality rate. Statistically significant reductions in risk were seen specifically for prostate, colorectal, and lung cancers.

field, feels that these three trials should not outweigh the piles of evidence that support beta-carotene's use in safe doses.

"If eating a carrot a day is safe, then supplementing up to the equivalent amount, about 20,000 IU, shouldn't be a problem," Dr. Anderson says.

Besides taking a multivitamin/mineral supplement, Dr. Anderson advises taking 10,000 IU of beta-carotene a day for general cancer protection. If you have a strong family history of cancer, or have already been diagnosed with some type of the disease, he suggests

Dr. Clark notes that further trials are needed to confirm these apparent beneficial effects of selenium supplementation. Dr. Anderson recommends getting selenium through a multivitamin containing at least 60 micrograms per day to protect against cancer. He advises people with cancer to consider taking 120 micrograms daily.

Selenium supplements are not recommended by the National Cancer Institute because there is a narrow margin between safe and toxic doses. People taking more than 100 micrograms of selenium a day should do so only under a doctor's supervision.

Colds

How to Make Them Less Common

A really bad cold can leave you feeling like you've been trampled by a rhinocerous. That would help explain how the guys in white lab coats came up with the term rhinovirus to describe the tiny organisms that cause about half of all common colds. (Coronaviruses—relax, it has nothing to do with Corona beer—are responsible for most of the rest.) You can catch one of these nasty buggers by inhaling virus-containing droplets (coughed or sneezed into the air by someone with a cold) or by rubbing your eyes or nose with contaminated fingers. Your hands can be infected by holding objects or shaking hands with people who carry the virus.

Once inside, the virus can eventually infect cells lining your nose or throat. An infected cell sends out signals to the rest of the body for help, and cold symptoms—such as nasal drip, sneezing, and phlegm-producing coughing—are unleashed to try to clear the virus out. This process usually takes about a week or so to run its course. Since there are hundreds of viruses out there, it's impossible to know exactly how long any particular one will last or even which symptoms it will produce.

Decrease Your Downtime

While there's no scientific evidence that vitamins and minerals can keep you from catching a cold, there are micronutrients that can cut the length and severity of one.

Here's what you need to know.

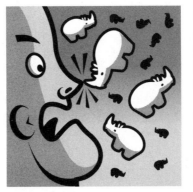

Make the zinc link. In a study done at the Cleveland Clinic Foundation in Ohio, 100 adult employees who were in the first 24 hours of their cold symptoms were asked to take a lozenge every 2 hours (except, naturally, when they were sleeping). The people were instructed to take the lozenges until all their symptoms went away. Without knowing who got which, the researchers gave half the sick people zinc gluconate lozenges and the other half placebos. The group that got the zinc gluconate had a whopping 42 percent reduction in the duration of their cold symptoms—an average of about 3.2 days shorter—compared to the group that got the dummy pills.

"It wasn't that they just felt better faster; their colds were completely gone. Statistically, the zinc gluconate lozenges worked significantly faster for cough, headache, hoarseness, nasal congestion, nasal drainage, and sore throat. All those got better faster, but the main thing is that the colds themselves went away more quickly," says Michael Macknin, M.D., senior investigator of the study. That's not to say that the virus was gone, but at least it wasn't creating havoc in the body.

There were a few side effects from the lozenges observed in Dr. Macknin's study. First, 80 percent of the people taking zinc gluconate lozenges reported a bad aftertaste. Second, 20 percent experienced some nausea. While Dr. Macknin is not ready to recommend zinc gluconate lozenges to the general public until there is more research supporting its benefits, he says that it's perfectly safe to try them if you're suffering from a cold. "Three out of the four members of my family will take it when they get a cold. Because of the bad taste, my daughter says she'd rather be sick," he says.

Reach for the right one. Remember that these exciting findings had nothing to do with zinc supplement pills—researchers were specifically examining zinc gluconate lozenges. There is no proof that zinc works to prevent a cold, so taking excessive doses is not recommended. Besides, large quantities of zinc taken for long periods of time can be dangerous, warns Dr. Macknin. It can cause decreased levels of copper in the body, which decreases the immune system's ability to fight off infections. Excessive amounts of zinc may also increase blood levels of low-density lipoprotein, or LDL, cholesterol (the bad kind) and decrease high-density lipoprotein, or HDL, cholesterol (the good kind).

You can get zinc gluconate lozenges at many stores that carry natural foods and homeopathic products, but be sure that you get the kind that works. Other forms of zinc lozenges have been studied, and while they did raise serum levels of the micronutrient in the body, they did not make colds go away faster, Dr. Macknin says. The type to look for contains zinc gluconate-glycine. "Rhinoviruses have canyons on their surfaces that seem to lock onto protrusions in the lining of the respiratory tract, then penetrate it. Theoretically, if you have the little zinc ions floating around, they plug up those canyons so that the rhinoviruses can't bind," he says.

And although combining zinc gluconate with ascorbic acid (vitamin C) might seem like a double-barrel cold blaster, the result is exactly the opposite. The popular antioxidant vitamin, while it may improve the taste, may actually bind up zinc, taking it out of the ionic state that makes it effective.

"You don't want to take a lozenge at the same time as you drink a glass of orange or grapefruit juice or swallow a supplement with vitamin C in it either. The citric acid in orange or grapefruit juice inactivates the lozenge, and the vitamin C makes it taste terrible," says Sabrina Novick, Ph.D., assistant professor of chemistry at Hofstra University in Hempstead, New York. Dr. Novick, along with her parents and study leaders, John C. Godfrey, Ph.D., and Nancy J. Godfrey, Ph.D., published the first investigation into zinc gluconate lozenges.

Cold-Eeze Lozenges is the only product that fits the bill right now, Dr. Novick says. Dr. John C. Godfrey teamed up with The Quigley Corporation to produce the patented product. If you can't find the lozenges in health food stores in your area, contact the distributor: The Quigley Corporation, Landmark Building, P.O. Box 1349, Doylestown, PA 18901.

Supplement with vitamin C.

Although it remains controversial in scientific circles, there is evidence that megadosing on vitamin C can help fight off the cold virus. A review conducted by a British researcher found that all the studies done since 1970 in which people were taking 1,000 milligrams or more of vitamin C a day to reduce the symptoms of their colds showed positive results, including one trial that reported a 72 percent reduction in the duration of cold symptoms. (Remember that the Daily Value for vitamin C is just 60 milligrams.) Check with your doctor before supplementing because intakes above 1,200 milligrams may cause diarrhea.

Three separate studies on men, led by Elliot Dick, Ph.D., retired professor of preventive medicine and chief of the respiratory virus research laboratory at the University of Wisconsin in Madison, showed that taking vitamin C before you get a cold also can be helpful.

In each study, half the men were given 500-milligram doses of vitamin C at breakfast, lunch, and dinner and before bed each day, for a total of 2,000 milligrams. The rest of the men got placebos. All pills were administered by researchers, just to make sure that the subjects took their prescribed dosages. After 3½ weeks, the men were gathered in a windowless room to play cards and be exposed to cold viruses. Although all of the men came down with colds, the vitamin C supplements helped weaken the effects.

Dr. Dick explains that when vitamin C levels are high, your white blood cells (natural defenders against invading microorganisms) are apparently re-invigorated, giving them more of the energy they need to neutralize a cold virus.

Diabetes

Playing against Type

Simply put, diabetes—a disease that affects some 7.2 million American men—occurs when you have too much sugar in your blood and insufficient or ineffective insulin. Insulin is a hormone that's released into the bloodstream by the pancreas and unlocks receptors on the outside of cells so that the simple sugar known as glucose can be used as energy or stored for future use. Diabetes comes in two forms: Type I, or insulin-dependent diabetes, and Type II, or non-insulin-dependent diabetes. Type I, which primarily strikes during childhood, occurs when the pancreas is damaged.

Type II accounts for 85 to 90 percent of diabetes in men. In this form the pancreas does produce insulin, but muscle cell receptors don't allow the glucose to get inside. The result is an accumulation of excessive amounts of sugar in the blood. Eventually, this can lead to artery, eye, kidney, and nerve damage. Complications can occur, resulting in such severe troubles as heart disease, blindness, amputation, and even death.

Eighty percent of men with Type II are overweight, so getting on weight-management and exercise programs should be the first steps for people diagnosed or at risk for the disease, says Christine Beebe, R.D., president of health care and education for the American Diabetes Association (ADA) and director of the Diabetes Center at St. James Hospital and Health Centers in Chicago Heights, Illinois.

The Antioxidant Link

Vitamin C, vitamin E, and beta-carotene have been linked to reduced risk of heart disease—a

major killer of men with diabetes. The ADA recognizes the potential benefits from antioxidants and promotes eating a healthy diet to get these nutrients. "One thing we can say about populations that consume high levels of fruits and vegetables is that they seem to have a lower risk for heart disease," Beebe says.

Weight loss is important to men with diabetes, but a low-calorie diet can create a new set of problems. "If I have a patient who is on a restricted diet (less than 1,600 calories per day) because he is trying to lose weight, for example, I might ask him to take a multivitamin/mineral supplement each day to ensure that he is meeting his needs," says Beebe.

Other experts in the field feel more strongly about the role that antioxidants can play in diabetes prevention and management. A study conducted by Dr. James Anderson of the University of Kentucky showed that vitamins C and E and beta-carotene delayed the oxidation of low-density lipoprotein (LDL) cholesterol that leads to hardening of the arteries. That's something that can lengthen a diabetic's life and allow him time to get his blood sugars under control.

In addition, vitamins C and E have been linked to reduced oxidative damage to proteins that can cause harm to the kidneys and eyes in diabetics, Dr. Anderson says.

"Over the years I became persuaded by the evidence that antioxidants were good, and that we weren't getting enough of them," says Dr. Anderson. He recommends that diabetics get 20,000 IU of beta-carotene (a precursor to vitamin A) and 800 IU of vitamin E once a day, plus 500 milligrams of vitamin C two times a day.

Check with your doctor before supplementing above 600 IU of vitamin E or 15,000 IU of vitamin A. Vitamin E supplements should be taken with the highest-fat meal of the day in order to be best absorbed. It's a good idea to

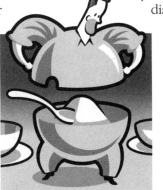

talk to your doctor before taking more than 400 IU of vitamin E daily because in big doses, the nutrient can interfere with anticoagulants. Extremely high doses may even interfere with the body's metabolism of vitamin K. Doses of vitamin C exceeding 1,200 milligrams a day can cause diarrhea in some people.

Aside from protecting us from heart disease, vitamin E may actually play a protective role against diabetes. "Laboratory studies on animals show that the use of vitamin E protects from several forms of experimental diabetes," Dr. Anderson says. Oxidative damage to the beta cells in the pancreas that make insulin contributes to the development of the disease. But research indicates that antioxidants—in particular, vitamin E—stop the damage before it is too late.

Mining for Protection

Certain minerals also may play a role in protecting against diabetes. Here are two of the most promising.

Chromium

A study done in China found that people who received chromium supplements improved their diabetes, perhaps because the mineral plays a role in the glucose tolerance factor that makes insulin work better, Beebe says. Unfortunately, this was only one study and the people in the study were probably chromium-deficient in the first place—something that isn't really a concern for most Americans, Beebe says.

While there's no good way to measure chromium deficiency, a multivitamin/mineral supplement is all you really need, Beebe says. "Some diabetic people will take chromium through brewer's yeast or some other form of supplementation. My suggestion to them is to try it for a couple of months to see if it works.

Keys to Health

Men with diabetes can do several things to control their disease, says Christine Beebe of the American Diabetes Association and St. James Hospital and Health Centers. Among them are the following:

- Maintain your proper body weight.
- Eat at least five servings of fruits and vegetables each day.
- Exercise regularly.
- Eat a high-fiber diet that focuses on unrefined carbohydrates instead of simple sugars.
- Use alcohol in moderation (no more than two drinks per day for men). If you take insulin, consult your physician first.

But if it doesn't, stop wasting your money," she says.

Dr. Anderson suggests that older people with diabetes should consider taking about 100 to 200 micrograms a day of chromium, either through brewer's yeast or chromium picolinate supplements.

If you are diabetic and want to try chromium supplements, tell your doctor. He may need to adjust your insulin dosage as your blood sugar levels drop.

Magnesium

If a person is not in good control of his diabetes, his magnesium levels may be lower than desirable, Beebe cautions. Preliminary research has indicated that low levels of magnesium may cause glucose intolerance, or vice versa.

Until further data are available on this connection, Beebe recommends getting the Daily Value of magnesium (400 milligrams). People with kidney problems should talk to their doctors first before beginning magnesium supplementation.

Diarrhea

A Way off Skid Row

Diarrhea is almost as uncomfortable to talk about as it is to suffer through. That's probably why we have so many slang terms for it—the runs, the trots, the skids, the undercover mud slide.

Physicians talk about diarrhea in more technical terms. Normal stool weighs somewhere around 100 grams, of which about half is water weight. Moderate diarrhea is about 400 grams, with water accounting for the added weight. Severe diarrhea is anything higher than that and can result in a person losing as much as 4 pints of fluid a day, says Peter Holt, M.D., chief of the division of gastroenterology at St. Luke's–Roosevelt Hospital Center and professor of medicine at Columbia University College of Physicians and Surgeons, both in New York City. Fortunately, you don't need to weigh the result to know if you have diarrhea. It usually comes on like a sudden avalanche down below, sometimes accompanied by abdominal pain. In an instant, the victim is sprinting for the nearest bathroom.

You may never know exactly what caused a particular case of the trots. "There are a million and one causes of diarrhea," says Joel B. Mason, M.D., assistant professor of medicine and nutrition at Tufts University School of Medicine in Boston. "Acute infectious diarrhea, what people call gastrointestinal flu, is usually related to a viral or bacterial infection. It is self-limiting and usually runs its course in several days to a week. The only immediate danger is the loss of fluids and electrolytes, including sodium, magnesium, potassium, and calcium."

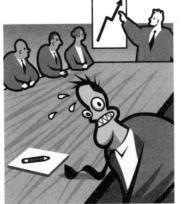

In the Belly of the Beast

Diarrhea can occur from either the colon or small intestine, Dr. Holt says. Diarrhea in the colon is not particularly troublesome. It usually only results in malabsorption of potassium and occasionally sodium, since little else of importance is absorbed there. When diarrhea strikes in the small intestine, however, malabsorption of many macronutrients and micronutrients—including vitamins as well as calcium, magnesium, potassium, and other electrolytes—can occur, he says.

"Diarrhea that comes as a result of a small-bowel disease can affect the absorption of many substances, since the small bowel is where these nutrients are digested," Dr. Holt says. If the diarrhea is prolonged, nutritional deficiencies and depletions can occur. The same is true with serious stomach or small-intestine operations or with diseases such as celiac sprue (an illness where gluten causes damage to the lining of the small intestine), ulcerative colitis (a condition of chronic inflammation and ulceration of the lining of the colon and rectum), Crohn's disease (a chronic inflammation of any part of the gastrointestinal tract), and HIV (human immunodeficiency virus).

"The issue of diarrhea most of the time is, 'What's the diagnosis?'—not what vitamin or mineral should a person take," Dr. Holt says. That's because if the illness causing the diarrhea is cured, the diarrhea goes away, too. In cases where there is no known or expedient remedy for the disease that is causing the diarrhea, doctors must determine where in the small intestine the problem is taking place because the location helps pinpoint which nutrients are being lost.

The next step is to fortify the patient's body with the missing nutrients through shots, supplements, or some other intervention. Chronic replacement of specific nutrients depends on the type of ailment and location of affected intestinal tissue, Dr. Holt says. For example, people who have had operations to remove the part of the small intestine called the ileum must have monthly vitamin B_{12} shots because they no longer have the ability to absorb the nutrient.

Doctors can determine where a chronic diarrhea problem is coming from by running a series of tests. Some tests check to see what nutrients aren't being absorbed. This is done by examining blood, stool, or small-intestine fluid samples. Other ways to examine the condition include x-ray and colonoscopy. Biopsies of the small intestine or colon also may be called for to determine what is causing the diarrhea.

Surviving the Short Term

Events of acute diarrhea that are caused by common viruses and bacteria are usually over within 12 to 72 hours. They aren't a real cause for alarm, Dr. Holt says. Only very young children, very old people, and those who are very ill to begin with are at any risk of harm during these brief stints. "Short-lived events of diarrhea rarely result in deficiencies or depletions of any essential vitamins or minerals in healthy adults," Dr. Holt says.

When you do come down with a case of acute diarrhea, here are a few simple things you can do to ensure against nutrient depletion and to encourage a speedy recovery, says Dr. Holt.

Go slow. If you are nauseous and vomiting, don't try fluids or foods just yet. Wait out the storm, then try drink some fluids.

Wash down the electrolytes. Since you are losing so much fluid in your diarrhea, you need to prevent dehydration. Drinking just water probably isn't enough, Dr. Holt says. You also need to replace electrolytes, the nutrients responsible for regulating many essential body

---

Call the Doctor

Dr. Peter Holt of St. Luke's–Roosevelt Hospital Center and Columbia University College of Physicians and Surgeons says that you should seek medical attention immediately if:

- **You have blood or pus in your diarrhea. These may be signs of a more serious infection or illness.**
- **You have diarrhea more than three days (more than 8 to 12 hours for young children and older people).**
- **You also have a fever or feel sluggish. These are indications that you are experiencing more than just acute infectious diarrhea.**
- **You show any signs of dehydration. These include a dry mouth and skin, very concentrated urine, and decreased frequency of urination.**

---

functions, including muscle movement, blood pressure, heart rate, and nerve impulses. Because your needs for electrolytes—especially sodium and potassium—are higher when you have diarrhea, drinking sports drinks, like Gatorade, can help replenish your stores. Start by slowly sipping about 4 ounces of a sports drink an hour. Some patients have difficulty tolerating these drinks, Dr. Holt says. He recommends diluting the beverage with water.

"The classic, old recommendation for people who had diarrhea was Coca-Cola because it has some potassium in it," Dr. Holt says. If you are drinking Coke, take it in the same way you would the sports drink.

Keep it bland, keep it small. If you have been sipping your fluids faithfully for about a day and the diarrhea seems to have slowed down, it's probably all right to try to eat something again, says Dr. Holt. Stick with carbohydrates that are mild, like plain pasta, bananas, white bread, or applesauce and keep the portions very small. If the runs stay away, gradually increase your portions. Once you can eat normal amounts again, it's probably okay to go back to your regular diet.

Eye Problems

Seeing Is Believing

Growing up, you must have heard it a thousand times: "Eat your carrots. They're good for your eyes." Skeptical of authority even at a young age, particularly where vegetables were concerned, you turned to the one source that you knew you could rely on for the unvarnished truth: Looney Toons. Sure enough, there was Bugs Bunny, the sharpest character in cartoon land, munching on carrots while he saw through the nefarious schemes of Elmer Fudd and Daffy Duck.

So it was that the connection between nutrition and vision was confirmed. It has taken scientists, who probably wasted their youth doing homework instead of watching cartoons, much longer to document the link. But they have found that what you eat might play an important role in two major age-related eye problems: cataracts and macular degeneration. Both are conditions that generally affect people after age 60 but in different ways.

Cataracts. The lens of the eye is mostly composed of protein. When everything's working well, the lens is crystalline clear. A cataract is the partial or complete clouding of the lens. The cloudiness begins to blur or dim vision, but a change in glasses can often correct the problem. Eventually, the extent of lost vision may make surgery an option. "Cataract surgery is the most commonly performed operation in the United States today," says Wayne Fung, M.D., an ophthalmologist and clinical professor of ophthalmology at California Pacific Medical Center in San Francisco, and a spokesman for the American Academy of Ophthalmology.

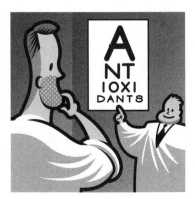

Implant surgery can replace the most damaged part of the lens with synthetic material. After that, any future cataracts can easily be cleared up with laser surgery, says Dr. Fung. These surgeries have a high success rate but are costly.

Macular degeneration. This affects the "heart" of the retina, the macula, the area that sends the brain fine details and color images. Age-related macular degeneration (ARMD) most often occurs in two forms: "dry" and "wet." The dry form is where gradual loss of contrasts between letters, or gradual fading of colors takes place as a result of the natural deterioration of the macular cells over many years of life, says Dr. Fung. The less common, wet form of ARMD can come on fairly abruptly, resulting from an invasion of newly sprouted blood vessels beneath the macula that can blur and distort images and straight lines. Unlike cataracts, the treatment of either form of ARMD is less successful.

Say "Eye" to Antioxidants

When it comes to exactly how nutrition plays a role in cataracts and ARMD, researchers and doctors don't know anything definite—yet. Antioxidants—specifically vitamins C and E and beta-carotene—have shown the most promise in several epidemiological and animal studies, Dr. Fung says.

Foods rich in antioxidants have been associated with lower risks of ARMD. In a study of 876 people with and without ARMD conducted by Johanna M. Seddon, M.D., at Harvard Medical School and by her colleagues around the country, people who reported consuming the highest amounts of carotenoids had a 43 percent lower risk for ARMD compared with those people who consumed the least.

"I recommend eating

beta-carotene-rich foods to my cataract and macular degeneration patients. I'd rather see them spend money on foods that are high in beta-carotene than on expensive supplemental products," says Dr. Fung. In addition to the beta-carotene and other antioxidants in produce, he says that patients will get the added benefits of fiber, which most people don't get enough of anyway.

Oxidation results in free-radical damage in the macula, which may be responsible for ARMD. Ultraviolet light, smoking, and a host of other causes may spark the oxidation. "When light energy is converted into nerve energy that is to be sent back to the vision center of the brain, the process occurs in the photoreceptors of the retina. We think that this photochemical reaction might generate free radicals that affect the macula, resulting in macular degeneration," Dr. Fung says. Antioxidants, which neutralize the free radicals, might be able to prevent or lessen this damage.

How this works is still a bit of a mystery. Dr. Fung explains that the free radicals damage the retinal pigment epithelium (RPE) layer of the macula. The theory is that if the RPE layer is protected, it can perform both nourishing and free-radical-removing functions that keep macular degeneration at bay. If this is true, antioxidants may be the key, says Dr. Fung. Antioxidants may work along the same principles for cataracts, only affecting the clear lens of the eye instead of the macula, Dr. Fung says.

"Oxidation is clearly an insult to the lens," says Allen Taylor, Ph.D., director of the Laboratory for Nutrition and Vision Research at the Jean Mayer U.S. Department of Agriculture Human Nutrition Research Center on Aging at Tufts University in Boston. The most frequent correlation between risk of cataract and nutrition is vitamin C, he says.

"We're very interested in a possible protective effect with vitamin C, since it is a water-soluble antioxidant and the lens is composed mostly of water and protein," Dr. Taylor says.

Smoke Gets in Your Eyes

Smoking has been linked repeatedly in studies to age-related macular degeneration and cataracts.

Like you really needed another reason to quit. Puffing tobacco results in free radical damage to the lens and macula. "I consider smoking to be a major risk factor for these diseases, no matter what your nutritional status. The evidence is just piling up against it," says Dr. Wayne Fung of California Pacific Medical Center.

Some animal studies show that vitamin C may have a protective effect, but these findings are not enough to make recommendations for humans.

What has yet to be determined is whether changing the levels of nutrients in our diets can actually alter our risk for these eye diseases. While some studies have indicated a relationship between low levels of antioxidant nutrients and risk for ARMD, for example, there is still no proof that high doses of the nutrient result in reduced risk, says Julie Mares-Perlman, Ph.D., assistant professor of ophthalmology and visual sciences at the University of Wisconsin Medical School in Madison. Dr. Mares-Perlman has been following approximately 2,000 people as part of a long-term, continuing study of the prevalence and risk factors for age-related eye diseases in the mid-size Wisconsin town of Beaver Dam.

Because more research needs to be done on the connection between antioxidants and age-related eye disease, Dr. Taylor says that it would be premature to recommend specific supplementing strategies. Anyone consuming the recommended five to nine servings a day of fruits and vegetables will cover most of the nutrients they need. Getting enough vitamin C, beta-carotene, and other carotenoids is easy enough to do through food, says Dr. Taylor. But taking a multivitamin/mineral supplement as an insurance policy may be beneficial.

Heart Disease

The News Is Simply FABB-ulous

The odds are stacked against us, guys. For a variety of reasons, ranging from heredity to bad habits, that Y chromosome we carry around is a marker for greatly increased heart attack risk. Men are more likely to die from heart disease than from anything else. It accounts for nearly half of all American male deaths, killing roughly half a million of us every year. And, yes: It is a guy thing. Before age 65, men suffer heart attacks at almost three times the rate of women.

By now, you know that you can cut your risk by not smoking; eating a low-fat, high-fiber diet; exercising at least three days a week; and effectively managing your stress levels. But if you're interested in tilting the odds even further in your favor, consider supplementing smartly with vitamins and minerals.

Be advised that not all experts in the field are ready to give supplementation blanket approval. "We do not yet have a clear consensus on supplements and won't until clinical trials prove their effectiveness. There is clear agreement, however, that eating a balanced diet with at least five servings of fruits and vegetables a day is important for heart health," says Ronald Krauss, M.D., head of the molecular medicine department, Lawrence Berkeley National Laboratory at the University of California, Berkeley, and chairman of the American Heart Association's Nutrition Committee.

Still, many experts are ready to give supplements the green light. One of the reasons is because heart disease risk doesn't just ride on your cholesterol and triglyceride numbers.

"Lipids are still an important factor in coronary artery disease, but there are other nutritional factors that can influence and help prevent disease as well," says Robert M. Russell, M.D., associate director of the Jean Mayer U.S. Department of Agriculture Human Nutrition Research Center on Aging at Tufts University in Boston. (For more information on lipids and nutrition, see High Cholesterol on page 116.)

The Homocysteine Chapel

The most exciting noncholesterol research relating to heart disease centers around one little amino acid in the blood called homocysteine. What makes amino acids important is that they are the building blocks of protein. But in the case of homocysteine, too much can mean trouble. It can be toxic to the blood vessel wall, allowing plaque to form, Dr. Russell says. In several studies, high blood homocysteine levels were strongly associated with higher risks for coronary artery disease.

Although researchers don't know exactly what causes elevated levels of homocysteine in the blood, they have made some interesting findings. Studies have drawn a connection between high homocysteine in the blood and inadequate levels of several B-complex vitamins. An examination of 1,401 men and women from the Framingham Heart Study found that when blood concentrations of folic acid, vitamin B_6, and vitamin B_{12} were low, homocysteine levels were higher. And moderate to high concentrations of the vitamins corresponded to lower homocysteine levels. Further, inadequate blood levels of one or more of these B vitamins appeared to contribute to 67 percent of the cases of high homocysteine.

While some people may be genetically susceptible to high homocysteine, many may simply have their diets to blame. "Research has shown us that if

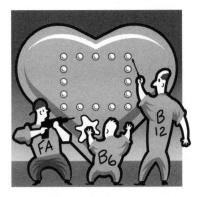

any or all of these vitamins are low in the body, then homocysteine will build up. And when you give these vitamins back to people with high levels, their homocysteine levels drop," Dr. Russell says. "A few years ago, no one would have ever suspected that water-soluble vitamins, such as folic acid, vitamin B_6, and vitamin B_{12} would play a role in the prevention of heart disease. But now we have evidence that they play a role through the homocysteine mechanism."

The Beatles may have been the Fab Four, but to protect your heart, you should remember the "FABB" Three: Folic Acid, B_6, and B_{12}.

"Folic acid seems the most likely candidate for lowering homocysteine, but since some people are responsive to vitamin B_6 and some to vitamin B_{12}, it's difficult to determine which B vitamin is at the root of the problem. I, as a general measure, recommend taking all three," says Dr. James Anderson of the University of Kentucky.

The Framingham Heart Study suggests that when folic acid levels drop below the Daily Value of 400 micrograms a day, homocysteine levels rise.

"If you are eating a healthy diet that includes at least five servings of fruits and vegetables a day, you should be able to reach homocysteine-lowering levels of the nutrient. If not, you should consider taking a multivitamin containing 100 percent of the Daily Value for folic acid," Dr. Russell says. Multivitamins also will give you levels of vitamins B_6 and B_{12} that are slightly higher than the Daily Value (2 milligrams and 6 micrograms, respectively), which seems to be all you need to have an effect on homocysteine.

Dr. Anderson suggests that if heart disease runs in your family, or if you have already been diagnosed with hardening of the arteries, your daily intake should be more.

Favor the Fighting Flavonoids

Fruits, vegetables, red wine, and green tea all provide the body with antioxidant compounds called flavonoids, which some research suggests may lower heart disease risks. In a study of elderly Dutch men, diets high in flavonoids were associated with a 68 percent lower heart attack death rate than diets low in the compounds, says Dr. James Anderson of the University of Kentucky. In another study of 5,000 people from 30 different Finnish communities, researchers found that people who consumed the most flavonoid-rich foods—primarily apples and onions—had the lowest rates of death from heart attack.

Research still needs to be done to see exactly how flavonoids work, but some experts believe that they counteract low-density lipoprotein (LDL) cholesterol, the bad stuff that causes plaque buildup on artery walls. In addition to eating lots of fruits and vegetables, Dr. Anderson drinks 2 or more cups of flavonoid-rich green tea a day and recommends that approach for others until further research is done.

These individuals, he advises, should take 1 milligram (1,000 micrograms) of folic acid, 25 milligrams of vitamin B_6, and 10 milligrams of vitamin B_{12} daily. One caution: Check with your doctor before supplementing folic acid above 400 micrograms because it can mask signs of a vitamin B_{12} deficiency.

Other Vitamins

The B-complex vitamins aren't the only players in the heart protection game. Research shows that vitamins E and C as well as beta-carotene may help keep your ticker ticking longer. Here's what you should know.

Vitamin E

Vitamin E helps keep your heart healthy in two ways: Its antioxidant powers help prevent low-density lipoprotein (LDL, the bad) cholesterol from oxidizing into plaque-forming guck on your artery walls, and the nutrient also serves as an anticoagulant. "It may work by having some interaction with the platelets in the blood, which are the cells that cause blood clotting. Vitamin E also works with vitamin K, which is necessary for the synthesis of various clotting factors," Dr. Russell says.

Regardless of which way vitamin E is working to lower heart disease risks, research from all over the world shows that it does the job effectively. Even in a study of more than 11,000 older folks, ages 67 to 105, conducted by researchers at the National Institute on Aging, use of vitamin E was associated with roughly a 40 percent reduction in coronary disease deaths, compared with nonuse of the supplement. That's after variables such as smoking history and use of alcohol were factored into the picture.

"Almost all the research that has been done on vitamin E points to much higher dosages than are possible with just a healthy diet," Dr. Russell says. Since a beneficial effect has been shown only with much higher amounts than the Daily Value of vitamin E—30 international units (IU)—supplementation is necessary, he says. That means that doctors and patients have to treat vitamin E like an over-the-counter medication, not a nutrient, says Dr. Russell.

Supplementation of 100 to 400 IU a day is considered effective and safe, Dr. Russell says. "If you are on another anticoagulant medication, like warfarin sodium (Coumadin) or aspirin, and plan to take more than 400 IU daily, you need to make your physician aware of it," he says. In very high doses (more than 800 IU),

Hearty Minerals

When it comes to matters of the heart, selenium may be just what the doctor ordered. The mineral selenium, found in grains, seafood, muscle meats, and Brazil nuts, may help activate the antioxidant gluthione peroxidase. This antioxidant discourages free radicals from boosting the artery-clogging low-density lipoprotein (LDL) cholesterol. In one Finnish study of 2,600 people, researchers found that people with blood selenium levels of about 103 micrograms per liter had a 60 percent lower risk of heart disease or cancer than people who were getting only about 60 micrograms.

Selenium also may work with vitamins C and E to help strengthen your cardiovascular system, says Dr. James Anderson of the University of Kentucky. He suggests that the average person take a daily multivitamin/mineral supplement with at least 60 micrograms of selenium and that people with heart disease, or who are at high risk for it, consider taking 120 micrograms of selenium daily. Check with your doctor before taking supplements of sele-

Dr. Russell warns that vitamin E appears to interfere with the body's metabolism of vitamin K—a nutrient necessary for the synthesis of blood-clotting materials.

Dr. Anderson recommends 800 IU of vitamin E to people who are at high risk for or who have evidence of heart disease. Check with your doctor before supplementing vitamin E above 600 IU daily. But don't think that popping vitamin E supplements is enough, he warns. It's effective only as part of a total lifestyle program that includes, among other things, healthy eating habits and regular exercise.

"I think that vitamin E is becoming a much more common physician recommendation and someday might be just as common as exercise. I tell my patients about it so that they can make up their own minds. I

nium over 100 micrograms. The Daily Value is 70 micrograms. Taking the supplement with a meal that has a bit of fat in it will aid in the absorption of selenium.

While you may want to add selenium to your diet, you definitely don't want to be an iron man. Some research has indicated that too much dietary iron may be associated with increased risk of heart disease in men. But a study of more than 4,000 men and women, conducted by the Centers for Disease Control and Prevention under the auspices of the National Institutes of Health, found that iron stores in the body did not relate to any risk of coronary heart disease at all.

Regardless of this one study, Dr. Anderson says that iron promotes the generation of free radicals, those troublesome molecules that make LDL cholesterol dangerous. It's best for men to limit their iron intake to 10 milligrams—an easy mark to meet with food. If you take a multivitamin/mineral supplement, look for one that contains no iron.

"I think that some of the problems that those studies found with beta-carotene stem from the kinds of dosages the subjects were given," Dr. Anderson says, adding that the extremely high supplemental doses used in those trials, nearly 17 times the Daily Value given every other day, resulted in far higher blood levels of beta-carotene than his recommendations do.

Dr. Anderson generally suggests that people get 10,000 IU of beta-carotene daily, the same amount he takes himself. By consuming five or more servings of fruits and vegetables a day, you should be able to meet that easily—one raw carrot alone puts you over the mark.

If you don't eat nutritiously, consider taking a multivitamin or beta-carotene supplement that meets these requirements.

Additional data indicate that beta-carotene and other carotenoids may prevent second heart attacks in people who have already survived one, Dr. Russell says.

also have recommended in several cases to take supplements of vitamin E," Dr. Russell says.

Beta-Carotene

The antioxidant beta-carotene, a precursor to vitamin A, was hailed as a very promising nutrient in research circles after several studies found that it was linked to reduced risk of heart disease. But it was dropped like a hot potato after several studies on humans using extremely high doses revealed either no effect on coronary artery disease or, as in the case of one Finnish study, even increased risk for heart disease and cancer. While some experts have backed off recommending supplements of any kind since, others are calling these studies a minor setback in the search for beta-carotene's potential.

Vitamin C

Although the research is less persuasive, vitamin C may be beneficial in the fight against heart disease, says Dr. Anderson. How it works is still unclear, but it seems that vitamin C might protect vitamin E from damage within the body.

"It appears that vitamin C can also raise high-density lipoprotein (HDL, the good) cholesterol levels, but we don't know if it will lower the risk of coronary artery disease in and of itself." Dr. Russell says.

"I think that vitamin C is where we will see the next major breakthrough in terms of increased Recommended Dietary Allowances," Dr. Anderson says. He advises that every adult get 250 milligrams of vitamin C twice daily, 500 milligrams twice daily if you have or are at high risk for coronary artery disease.

High Blood Pressure

Get Down with Minerals

For decades, sodium and high blood pressure have gone together like salt and pepper. If you had high blood pressure, the doctor would tell you to go easy on the salt (also known as sodium chloride). Like most things in life these days, though, it's not that simple anymore.

Sure, sodium may still be a factor for some guys with high blood pressure. But the latest research shows that other minerals play key roles in the equation that equals 120/80 and below (healthy blood pressure readings) or 140/90 and above (potentially dangerous levels).

Just a quick refresher if you haven't had your blood pressure checked lately: The first number, the systolic blood pressure, is a reading that measures the maximum force going away from the heart. The second number, the diastolic pressure, measures the minimum force of blood at the end of the heartbeat. These figures are important tools in determining your risk for stroke, heart attack, and kidney disease, so you should have your physician check your blood pressure at least once a year, says Edward Saltzman, M.D., medical director of the Obesity Center at the New England Medical Center and scientist at the Jean Mayer U.S. Department of Agriculture Human Nutrition Research Center at Tufts University School of Medicine in Boston. If your numbers are on the high side—formally known as hypertension—minerals may help you control them. Here's what you need to know.

Sodium

Because of how your body handles it, if you take in too much sodium, your body will hold on to more liquid to give the sodium something to swim in. This excess liquid makes the blood swell to a greater volume, and that causes your heart to work overtime, trying to pump all the blood through your system.

Even though some research has questioned whether salt is really to blame for hypertension in our diets, most experts agree that too much of it is bad news for sodium-sensitive individuals. "Sodium is one mineral that has shown a definite connection to hypertension in that too much can raise blood pressure," says Dr. Ronald Krauss of the Lawrence Berkeley National Laboratory at the University of California and the American Heart Association.

But there are generally two schools of thought when it comes to who needs to watch their sodium, says Dr. Saltzman. One school believes that everyone should have a low-sodium diet. That's because, regardless of whether a person actually develops high blood pressure with sodium, the mineral tends to elevate levels. Dr. Saltzman says that physicians in this corner of the debate feel that the lower your blood pressure, the less likely you are to have a stroke or a heart attack. So everyone should limit their sodium intake to 2,400 milligrams or less per day—period.

The other school of thought believes that only those people whose intakes of sodium seem to signal elevated blood pressure should care about how much sodium they eat or drink. The rest of the population doesn't need to be so careful. There's just one catch: The only practical way to identify a sodium-sensitive person is to limit his sodium consumption and see if his blood pressure comes down. "Often, when a person comes in and is newly diagnosed as hypertensive, the first thing he is told to do is lose any excess weight and decrease his dietary salt," Dr. Saltzman says. If the patient follows those instructions, it may not be clear if the shed pounds or the reduced salt did the trick, at least in the beginning.

Magnesium

Magnesium has shown moderate benefits in lowering high blood pressure in some studies, says Dr. Saltzman. One such study was conducted in Sweden on 71 people with mildly elevated blood pressures who were not taking any hypertension medications. Researchers found that giving magnesium supplements to folks who had low levels of the mineral appeared to reduce their blood pressure readings by several points.

A few points are enough to make a difference to a borderline hypertensive person, but they are not a big deal to someone with a bigger blood pressure problem, Dr. Saltzman says. "While some trials have shown benefits from taking magnesium supplements, it's just too early to know if there is any consistency to these findings," he says.

The American Heart Association is not ready to advocate magnesium, or any other mineral, as a significant factor in lowering blood pressure, Dr. Krauss says.

Dr. Saltzman suggests that getting your Daily Value's worth (400 milligrams) is a good idea, however. Dark green, leafy vegetables; whole grains; fish; legumes; and nuts are good sources of magnesium. Adult men seem to be able to get enough of this mineral from their diets, so supplements aren't necessary.

Potassium

To keep sodium levels from getting too high, the body also needs other minerals. One such nutrient is potassium, which helps clear your bloodstream of excess sodium. To make matters worse, a shortage of potassium can cause your body to hold on to more sodium. "In studies where diets of people who have

lower blood pressures are assessed, they tend to be higher in potassium as well as magnesium and calcium," says Dr. Saltzman. While some believe that potassium supplements may lower blood pressure, results of intervention trials have only shown moderate and inconsistent effects, he says.

"If you have a low dietary intake, or a deficiency, you are more likely to reap the benefit from increasing your potassium supplies than someone who gets enough of the mineral already," Dr. Saltzman says. The Daily Value for potassium, 3,500 milligrams, is all you need to keep you out of the deficiency doghouse. All the epidemiological studies supporting potassium as a blood pressure reducer have examined food intake, not supplements, says Dr. Saltzman. So sticking with food is your best bet. These foods include bananas, potatoes, yams, raisins, and a host of other fruits and vegetables and dairy products.

Apart from people on medications that lower potassium, supplements have not proved to be worth investing in, says Dr. Saltzman. Megadosing on potassium supplements is definitely out of the question. "If you exceed your body's ability to excrete potassium, it can cause fatal heart arrythmias," he cautions. People who have diabetes or kidney problems, or who are taking anti-inflammatory drugs, potassium-sparing diuretics (water pills), ACE (angiotensin converting enzyme) inhibitors, or heart medications should not supplement potassium without medical supervision.

Calcium

Very preliminary research has indicated that calcium may have a role in keeping blood pressure in check. "It may work with potassium somehow, or there may even be an independent effect of calcium. These ideas are very sketchy, at best, at this point," says Dr. Saltzman. Even if the research isn't very strong, he notes, this just shows another good reason to get your bone-protecting 1,000 milligrams of calcium each day.

High Cholesterol

High Noon in the Heartland

Today's topic: Is low-density lipoprotein, which goes by LDL for short, born to be bad? Or is it just the company it keeps?

It's the old question of nurture versus nature, applied to cholesterol. For years, LDL cholesterol has been the guy in the black hat, cast as the artery-clogging villain in the gunfight for your heart. Its brother, high-density lipoprotein, or HDL, has played the guy in the white hat, the sheriff who keeps your arteries safe by running LDL cholesterol out of Dodge. It turns out that it's not quite that black and white.

Both forms of cholesterol are soft, fatlike substances transported in the blood. In order to float through your bloodstream, cholesterol needs a coating of protein. This coating is called—you guessed it, pardner—lipoprotein. LDL cholesterol only turns mean when it becomes oxidized in the blood. That process sets loose destructive molecules called free radicals, which damage the blood vessel and artery walls, making it easier for plaque to form on them. That's what clogs your arteries.

If you can prevent LDL cholesterol from oxidizing, you can prevent—and even reverse—hardening of the arteries, which, in turn, can lead to heart attacks and strokes, says Dr. James Anderson of the University of Kentucky. That's where antioxidants come in. And vitamins E and C are just what the doctor ordered, he says.

Vitamin E: Radical Action Hero

So what would LDL cholesterol be like if it didn't hang out with those rampaging free

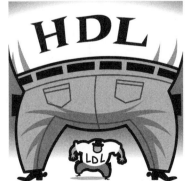

radicals? "If you can prevent the LDL cholesterol from being oxidized, then it doesn't have as damaging a property," says Dr. Robert M. Russell of Tufts University. In effect, LDL might be a nicer cholesterol if it could be sheltered from oxidation. That's what vitamin E tries to do.

Studies on both animals and humans have shown that high levels of vitamin E in the blood have been strongly associated with reduced coronary artery diseases and deaths, Dr. Anderson says.

Vitamin E attacks the free radicals, destroys them, then lets the leftover particles wash away in the bloodstream, he says. This prevents a whole series of events that can lead to heart attacks and strokes.

"Alpha-tocopherol, a compound in vitamin E, is responsible for about 90 percent of the antioxidant factor that goes to work on LDL cholesterol in the blood," Dr. Anderson says. Other vitamin E compounds, such as gamma-tocopherol, are being investigated, but Dr. Anderson says that it's too early to know how effective they might be in the fight against heart disease.

It's next to impossible to get all the vitamin E you need from food. That's where supplements come into play. According to both Dr. Russell and Dr. Anderson, 400 international units (IU) of vitamin E—which is more than 13 times the Daily Value of 30 IU—is a safe and effective dose. If you already have heart disease, or are at very high risk for it, Dr. Anderson suggests taking 800 IU of vitamin E daily.

If you plan to take levels higher than 600 IU, discuss it with your doctor first. Doses above that mark can interfere with anticoagulating medications, and doses higher than about 800 IU can disturb your body's vitamin K metabolism.

Note: Supplementing with vitamin E isn't a cure-all. For total heart health, the American Heart Association recommends a lifestyle program that includes losing excess weight, quitting smoking, cutting down the fat (especially saturated fat) and cholesterol in your diet, increasing your dietary fiber intake, eating five to nine servings of fruits and vegetables a day, and exercising at least 30 minutes three times a week.

Vitamin C: Best Supporting Actor

If vitamin E gets an Oscar for its performance as a free-radical basher, the Academy Award for best supporting actor would have to go to vitamin C. Vitamin E is constantly being repaired by vitamin C in the blood. Because of this, vitamin E can work effectively at controlling LDL cholesterol oxidation, Dr. Anderson says.

Vitamin C might have cholesterol-tapping functions of its own, too. Researchers measured levels of vitamin C in the blood (from either foods or supplements) in 827 men and women participating in the Baltimore Longitudinal Study on Aging. The study was conducted by the National Institute on Aging in Bethesda, Maryland, to find out how vitamin C affects HDL cholesterol levels. The study found that, up to a certain dietary level, the more vitamin C people got, the higher their HDL levels were. In women, 215 milligrams a day seemed to be the optimum amount. In men, 346 milligrams appeared to be the maximum.

"It appears that vitamin C can raise HDL cholesterol levels, but we don't know if it will lower the risk of coronary artery disease in and of itself," Dr. Russell says. Until further evidence regarding this nutrient is found, exercise remains the best proven way to raise your HDL

Go Slow with Niacin

Warning: Taking slow-release niacin as a cholesterol-lowering treatment is risky business. While niacin does lower cholesterol (even the low-density lipoprotein kind that clogs arteries), troubling side effects have doctors and patients concerned. The complications are great enough that about half the people who take slow-release niacin do not continue with the nutritional supplement as a long-term therapy.

Researchers at Virginia Commonwealth University, Medical College of Virginia School of Medicine, in Richmond, and at Pennsylvania State University College of Medicine in Hershey teamed up to examine slow-release niacin. They found that this form of niacin can create liver enzyme levels three times higher than normal in half the people taking the treatment. Twenty-five percent of them actually showed symptoms of liver malfunction, including fatigue, nausea, and loss of appetite. Fortunately, once off the niacin, their livers returned to normal after about a month.

The researchers concluded that the slow-release niacin and the immediate-release form should be taken only under a doctor's supervision.

levels. The Daily Value for vitamin C is 60 milligrams. That's enough to prevent the deficiency disease scurvy, says Dr. Anderson; but it does nothing to provide cholesterol benefits. He recommends that people consume a healthy diet with lots of vitamin C–rich fruits and vegetables and that they take a 250-milligram supplement twice daily. If you have high cholesterol or heart disease already, Dr. Anderson recommends that you take 500 milligrams of vitamin C twice daily. At these levels, the water-soluble vitamin is considered quite safe.

HIV

Getting the Nutrients You Need

If you test positive for the human immunodeficiency virus (HIV), one of the first calls that you should make is to a nutritionist. Why? Even if you show no symptoms and religiously follow a balanced diet, the virus probably is robbing your body of key nutrients, causing deficiencies in a slew of vitamins and minerals.

A study at the University of Miami of 112 men who were HIV-positive found that 67 percent had at least one nutrient deficiency, while 36 percent had more than one. Thirty percent were deficient in vitamin B_6, 30 percent in zinc, 20 percent in vitamin E, 16 percent in vitamin A, and 11 percent in vitamin B_{12}.

Yet, none of these men exhibited any symptoms—fatigue or memory loss, for example—of nutritional deficiency, and most were eating diets that provided all the Recommended Dietary Allowances (RDAs). Many also were taking supplements. But when vitamin B_{12} was measured, only those men taking 25 times the RDA demonstrated even adequate levels.

The connection between nutrition and HIV—the virus that destroys the immune system and causes AIDS—is complicated and still evolving, so seeking professional help immediately is vitally important, says Mehry Safaeian, R.D., clinical dietitian at the University of Pittsburgh Medical Center. "A nutritional program can aid in keeping your immune cell counts high," says Safaeian, who has been working with people with HIV/AIDS since 1990. "But we have to begin to fight the disease with nutrition as soon as possible because once the disease starts to take its toll, it's much harder to fight."

Get with the Program

A newly diagnosed patient should find a clinical nutritionist who has at least a master's-level degree in dietetics and nutrition (a certified nutrition specialist will have a C.N.S. after his or her name), and preferably specializes in working with AIDS and HIV-positive patients, says Shari Lieberman, C.N.S., Ph.D., an HIV/AIDS clinical nutritionist and co-author of The Real Vitamin and Mineral Book.

"Ask if they have some of the current nutrition science studies on HIV/AIDS that you could look at. Ask them if they see a lot of AIDS and HIV-positive patients. Ask them a lot of questions. If they are worth going to, they won't mind answering you or suggesting someone else to call," Dr. Lieberman says.

It helps to do your homework in advance, but self-diagnosis isn't a good idea, no matter what promising information you've read. As the University of Miami study shows, you could be doing everything nutritionally correct and still have deficiencies in several vitamins and minerals. And some nutrients, such as zinc and iron, can hamper the immune system if they are taken in excessive amounts, Safaeian says. As an example of how confusing things can get, consider the research on selenium. It's been found in low levels in HIV patients, indicating that they need more than normal doses for good immune system function. But it's also been suggested that excessive doses of the mineral may actually feed the HIV virus. If getting the right amounts of vitamins and minerals sounds like it can be tricky for people who are HIV-positive, that's because it is.

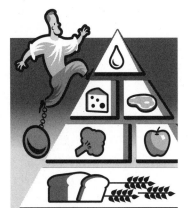

Turning the Double Play

The American Dietetic Association (ADA) says that getting 100 to 200 percent of the RDAs for vitamins and minerals is safe for people who are HIV-positive. A multivitamin/mineral supplement combined with a very nutrient dense diet is the way the ADA suggests to get these increased levels.

There are many reasons why HIV-positive people need to boost their intake of nutrients, says Keith-Thomas Ayoob, R.D., Ed.D., spokesman for the ADA in Chicago, director of nutrition services at the Rose F. Kennedy Children's Evaluation and Rehabilitation Center, and assistant professor of pediatric medicine at Albert Einstein College of Medicine, both in New York City. Often, complications and symptoms of the disease, such as vomiting, diarrhea, anorexia, or nausea, can cause malabsorption of certain nutrients. Drugs to treat the disease or its complications also can affect absorption or the need for various nutrients. A clinical nutritionist should work with a patient's doctor to determine the best nutritional course of action.

However, some experts who work in the field believe that the ADA's recommendations are too general. Dr. Lieberman, who has worked with HIV and AIDS patients since the beginning of the epidemic back in the mid-1980s, is one of them. She gives presentations all over the United States demonstrating the need for more radical nutritional programs to control the virus.

"People with this disease need more specific nutritional direction than simply doubling every vitamin RDA. There is a wealth of research data on specific nutrients, some of which do not even have an RDA, that demonstrate antiviral and immune-enhancing effects in this population," Dr. Lieberman says. "In terms of specific nutrients, antioxidants reduce oxidative stress and are antiviral at high doses. Some of these include beta-carotene, vitamin C, glutathione, N-acetylcysteine, and coenzyme Q_{10}, as well as other vitamins, minerals, and herbal preparations that are used to combat the disease by many knowledgeable practitioners. Acidophilus supplements are important to prevent bacteria, parasites, and other intestinal pathogens."

Because every patient will have different symptoms and progression of the disease, nutrients should be monitored by a clinical nutritionist at these high therapeutic doses. If it's something that patients want to try, Dr. Lieberman says that they shouldn't stop looking around until they find a nutritionist who is knowledgeable.

Fine-tuning the nutritional program for each patient is really what it comes down to with HIV. "As a starting point, consider a multivitamin with minerals that provides 100 percent of the RDA twice a day. Supplements should be taken with food and with plenty of water to help in its breakdown," says Safaeian.

Weight Up

"The first concern for people with HIV or full-blown AIDS is eating enough, period," Dr. Ayoob says. Wasting syndrome, a devastating side effect of HIV that results in rapid and severe weight loss, increases the body's need for calories and protein.

Dr. Ayoob has seen the need for protein increase to as much as 50 percent more than what is normally considered necessary. Everything from chronic low-grade fevers (which increase the caloric need 7 percent for every 1°F above normal body temperature) to minor infections can increase the need for calories, Dr. Ayoob says.

According to Dr. Lieberman, people with full-blown AIDS need at least 2 grams of protein per kilogram of body weight, which is twice the average person's requirements—or more like the amount needed by world-class bodybuilders and athletes.

High-fat sources of protein should not be considered for an HIV diet, however, because they have been shown to lower the body's immunity and increase the oxidation process, says Dr. Lieberman.

"It is also imperative that these people engage in an exercise and weight-lifting program," Dr. Lieberman says. "You can't preserve muscle mass without lifting weights."

Prostate Cancer

*Surprising Findings Offer
New Hope*

For an organ the size of a walnut, the prostate can cause huge health problems. Although prostate cancer targets mainly men over age 50, it's never too early to start thinking about how to reduce your chances of developing the disease. Caught early, prostate cancer can be stopped cold 91 percent of the time. Because it shows no symptoms until it's serious, the American Cancer Society recommends that all men over age 40 should get yearly checks.

First, get a yearly digital rectal exam, in which a doctor feels the prostate with a gloved finger to detect irregularities. This should begin at age 40. Second, get a blood test that measures prostate-specific antigen (PSA), a prostate-produced protein whose levels rise when the gland has a problem. For men over 50, the American Cancer Society recommends this blood test annually. High-risk men such as African-Americans and men who have a family history of prostate cancer should start both types of annual testing at age 40.

While testing is certainly important, scientists have uncovered intriguing evidence that certain nutrients may play a role in preventing prostate cancer.

Passing the Folic Acid Test

By age 50 or so, a man's prostate will most likely develop 10 to 1,000 cancerous cells, says Dr. Warren Heston of Memorial

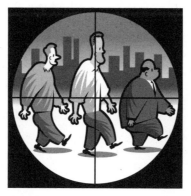

Sloan-Kettering Cancer Center. It's like a breeding ground for cancer. If this microscopic area does not expand or spread, then prostate cancer as a disease will not develop. If, for whatever reason, the lesion does grow, full-blown prostate cancer develops.

It now appears that folic acid may play a key role in determining whether cancer develops. This B vitamin—known as folate when it comes naturally from food—can diffuse into healthy prostate membrane cells. The trouble comes when there is a lot of the enzyme folate hydrolase in the prostate. Folate hydrolase may block folic acid from being glutamylated. Glutamylation prevents folic acid from being able to leak back out of a cell. This puts the prostate at substantial risk to develop 'localized folate deficiency,' which acts in concert with cancer-causing agents to develop cancers. Folate-deficient cells are more susceptible to cancer mutations, Dr. Heston says.

"Is prostate tissue at risk for folate deficiency due to an excess of folate hydrolase? That's what we need to find out," says Dr. Heston.

Because the prostate has too much folate hydrolase, Dr. Heston thinks that obtaining higher amounts of folic acid in the diet might turn out to be useful in controlling the onset of prostate cancer. "However, that might be a two-edged sword, because even though the prostate develops malignant cells, prostate cancers are often very slow growing. It is not certain whether high folic acid supplementation would increase the rate of tumor growth, and it is one of the reasons why I'm cautious of recommending very high supplementation of folic acid to anybody," he says.

Dr. Heston consciously tries to get more folate in his daily diet, and he takes a multivitamin/mineral supplement with 100 percent of the Daily Value for folic acid (400 micrograms). Foods that contain folate include vegetables, beans, fruits, whole grains, and fortified breakfast cereals.

And keep in mind that vitamins B_6 and B_{12} help folic acid do its job better. "It's like a car being tuned up: You want to make sure that everything, not just one part of the engine, is running smoothly," says Dr. Heston. A good multivitamin should help take care of this.

Protecting the Prostate

Scientists are looking at the potential of other vitamins and minerals to protect your prostate. Here are the most promising areas.

Vitamin E

In lung cancer studies examining the effects of beta-carotene and vitamin E, an unexpected discovery was made. "Interestingly, even though it wasn't protective against lung cancer, vitamin E given to patients—with and without beta-carotene—was associated with a 60 to 70 percent decrease in prostate cancer," Dr. Heston says. "Given as a supplement to those individuals, it did look like it was having an impact on the number of patients developing prostate cancer within the time frame of the trial."

It is not yet clear whether the nutrient exerts its effect on an unidentified receptor in the prostate, or whether it is having these beneficial effects by its known antioxidant effects, Dr. Heston says.

The vitamin E dosages in those studies were many times higher than the current Daily Value of 30 international units (IU), says Dr.

Too Much of a Good Thing

The way that zinc has been talked about, you'd think that the prostate gland was one big, solid mass of the mineral. Zinc is an important part of a healthy prostate, and studies have shown that inflammation can decrease the stores of the nutrient in the prostate tissue. So shouldn't all men be taking more of it?

"I would say that supplementation might not be necessarily helpful," says Dr. Warren Heston of Memorial Sloan-Kettering Cancer Center. "Everyone knows that zinc is in the prostate and that it has a role in prostate health, but nobody knows how to get more dietary zinc into the gland."

The thing to remember about zinc, says Dr. Heston, is that your body has a feedback system for the mineral. If you are kicking in a certain amount, and your body assumes that it has had enough, it will just turn off the absorption. You can overdo it with zinc, a mineral that can be toxic in very high doses. Too much zinc—levels between 25 and 30 milligrams—can also cause anemia and immunity problems, so doses above 15 milligrams should be taken under medical supervision. Individuals with impaired renal function may be more susceptible to toxicity and should consult their physician regarding their maximum dosage.

If you're eating well or taking a multivitamin/mineral supplement with zinc, Dr. Heston says, you're doing just about all you can do with the mineral. Even if you have an inflamed prostate, what you need to do is address what is causing the inflammation. Correct what's going on to irritate the prostate, and the zinc levels should return to normal, Dr. Heston says.

Heston. Ongoing trials are now focusing on giving about 800 IU of alpha-tocopherol (the compound in vitamin E that appears to have the greatest anti-cancer benefits) daily to men. "At this level, it's strong enough to act like a medication rather than a nutrient but still well below toxic amounts," Dr. Heston says. It's still too early to recommend taking vitamin E to all men, he notes. However, taking 400 IU daily—the same safe amount recommended by many doctors for heart disease prevention—may be beneficial for men with troublesome PSA readings, Dr. Heston says. If you are taking anticoagulant medications, talk to your doctor before supplementing with vitamin E.

Selenium

In a study led by Dr. Larry Clark of the Arizona Cancer Center, 1,312 people with a history of skin cancer were given either 200 micrograms of high-selenium yeast (a supplement) or a placebo over the course of 10 years. While skin cancer did not seem to be influenced, a significant reduction in risk was seen for prostate cancer.

While he feels that further research needs to be done before selenium supplementation can be promoted for prostate cancer prevention, Dr. Heston says that taking a multivitamin that includes selenium is safe and acceptable. High doses—100 to 200 micrograms—can be toxic and should only be taken under medical supervision.

Lycopene

There's a chemical in fruits and vegetables—especially tomatoes—called lycopene that may offer prostate cancer protection. Actually, lycopene comes from a good anti-cancer family. It's a carotenoid, like beta-carotene, and one of a growing number of phy-

---

Stay on the Sunny Side

Puzzled by the fact that men living in the northern third of the United States develop more prostate cancer than those in the Sun Belt, researchers turned to vitamin D, a nutrient your body manufactures from sunlight that it absorbs through the skin. Studies confirmed their suspicion on a biological level: According to recent research, men with higher levels of vitamin D in their blood are less likely to develop prostate cancer.

Researchers believe that darker men—including Asian-, Native-, and African-Americans—may be especially susceptible to the vitamin D deficiencies because their skin requires more sunlight to manufacture the nutrient. As a result, experts say that dark-skinned men would be well-advised to spend about 20 minutes a day in the sun. Because of the risk of skin cancer, most experts suggest that fair-skinned men get their D primarily in the form of fortified milk. Nutritionists believe that the calcium in milk might boost vitamin D's efficacy. For an extra mineral wallop, mix ¼ cup of nonfat dry milk into a cup of regular skim milk. This dry addition gives the drink a richer taste, and just two glasses a day deliver 90 percent of your daily required intake of vitamin D.

---

tochemicals in produce that researchers think might help fight off cancer, says Dr. James Anderson of the University of Kentucky.

A study of 47,849 men has shown a link between eating a lot of tomatoes, especially tomato sauce cooked with a little olive oil, and lower risk of prostate cancer. Compared with men who ate no tomato sauce, men who ate even as little as two servings a week had a 34 percent reduction in risk for prostate cancer. Researchers theorize that the cooking process and the touch of olive oil in the sauce seem to enhance the absorption of lycopene.

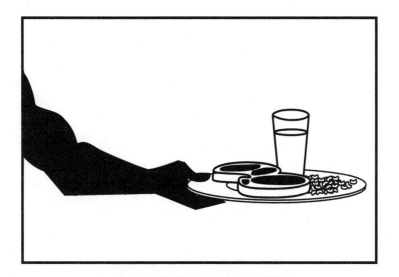

Part Five

Everyday Vitality

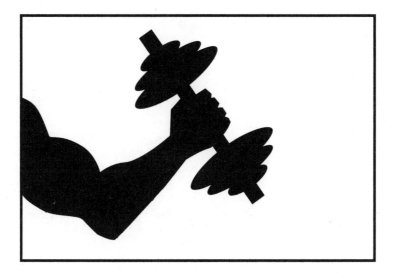

Enjoying Great Sex

Getting a Lift from Chemistry

You've dimmed the lights and lit enough candles to start a bonfire. A light, yet fruity chardonnay—her favorite—chills while the sumptuous gourmet meal you cooked (okay, bought at the deli counter of your grocery store) awaits on your wedding china.

When she walks through the door and gets a load of this spread, a night of great sex is virtually assured, right? As a matter of fact, you may have forgotten something—and it's not your notes from Men Are from Mars, Women Are from Venus. It's your vitamins and minerals.

To put it another way: You've done a masterful job of creating the right atmosphere for sexual chemistry to flourish. John Gray, Ph.D., author of the Mars and Venus books, would be proud. But you may have forgotten about your own personal chemistry.

Don't get the wrong idea. There's not a lot of proof that you'll turn into the Marathon Man simply by gobbling a handful of pills from the health food store—no more than you could transform Rosie O'Donnell into Cindy Crawford by sending her to the hairdresser. But there's increasing evidence that several key nutrients can help fend off male sexual problems like erectile dysfunction and infertility.

"Although the appropriate studies haven't yet been done, if we can apply what we know to be true about protecting and preserving the heart to the penis— with the right combination of exercise, eating habits, and nutrients—then one could expect the same positive results," says E.

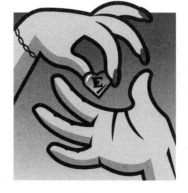

Douglas Whitehead, M.D., director of the Association for Male Sexual Dysfunction and associate clinical professor of urology at the Albert Einstein College of Medicine of Yeshiva University, both in New York City.

Here's the latest scoop on what you need to know to make sure that the big night comes out the way you planned.

Flow Motion

In a less enlightened era—pre-ESPN— lots of so-called experts thought that problems like erectile dysfunction were beyond the healing hands of medicine. One day in your mid-fifties, you'd wake up and discover that Sergeant Stiffman can no longer salute. And, short of some bizarre, painful medical procedure—penile prosthesis anyone?—that was the end of your sex life. Of course, this also occurred at a time when such problems were called impotence and you were more likely to lie down in front of a moving car than actually let anyone know that you were suffering from it.

Times have definitely changed for the better. For one thing, there are multiple all-sports channels broadcasting 24 hours a day. But more important, the experts better understand what can impair your penis. Research shows that nearly 80 percent of all men over age 50 with erectile dysfunction have vascular problems like cardiovascular disease, coronary artery disease, or diabetes.

One South Carolina study, for example, showed that erectile problems were 83 percent more likely in men with total cholesterol levels higher than 240 milligrams per deciliter than among those with levels under 180 milligrams per deciliter. Many of the guys in the study were college graduates who worked in white-collar or professional jobs.

"What actually happens

Sperm Wails

Over the past few decades, a growing number of experts have found evidence that men's sperm levels have dropped dramatically around the world.

One possible culprit is toxicity from industrial pollution in the form of the heavy metals lead, aluminum, and cadmium. "If you can believe it, I've found lead in seminal plasma, and that definitely decreases sperm viability—the amount of live sperm you have," says Earl Dawson, Ph.D., associate professor in the department of obstetrics and gynecology at the University of Texas Medical Branch at Galveston. "Aluminum is everywhere, too. Heck, everything you buy is in aluminum containers, so it's practically impossible not to have it in your system."

Although experts are divided over the cause and treatment, Dr. Dawson says that there are some do-it-yourself techniques for protecting your plumbing from this so-called toxic onslaught.

See if vitamin C makes a difference. Vitamin C, also called ascorbic acid, tops the list of nutrients that protect sperm because it has a "detoxifying effect" on many chemicals, says Dr. Dawson. In one study, Dr. Dawson divided 75 young male smokers into three groups. One group got a placebo, another got 200 milligrams of vitamin C daily for a month, the third took 1,000 milligrams of vitamin C daily for a month. The higher the men's vitamin C levels rose, the greater the protection they received against the sperm-damaging effects of nicotine.

"Most toxic substances are what are called oxidizing agents. The smallest amount kills bacteria, sperm, anything. But vitamin C counteracts this very well," says Dr. Dawson. He recommends taking 1,000 milligrams of ascorbic acid a day: 500 milligrams in the morning and 500 milligrams in the afternoon at supper time, or a quart of orange juice. The Daily Value of vitamin C is 60 milligrams, about the amount found in a medium-size orange. Why does Dr. Dawson recommend so much? For one thing, your body quickly removes excess vitamin C from your system, so you literally have to fill up every day to keep your tissues saturated.

Call on calcium. Calcium has long been used to defend against the ravages of lead by helping to remove it from your body, says Dr. Dawson. For protection, all you need to do is get the Daily Value of 1,000 milligrams—the same amount found in two 8-ounce glasses of skim milk and a cup of yogurt. "It's not a cure-all, but it should help," he says.

Zap it with zinc. While it's debatable whether a zinc deficiency can cause erectile dysfunction, men who don't get enough zinc have less ejaculate, according to a study authored by Curtiss Hunt, Ph.D., research biologist at the U.S. Department of Agriculture–Agricultural Research Service Grand Forks Human Nutrition Research Center in North Dakota. As zinc intake fell from more than 10 milligrams per day to just above 1 milligram, the amount of ejaculate dropped by nearly one-third. The Daily Value is 15 milligrams.

is that the arterial walls narrow, and so the velocity or the amount of the blood that can move through the artery leading to the penis is decreased," says L. Dean Knoll, M.D., director of research at the Center for Urological Treatment and Research in Nashville. "And when the amount of blood is decreased, you can't fill the spaces in the body of the penis."

"It's not unusual for the first sign of vascular disease to actually show up as impotence," says Dr. Whitehead. "It's literally a symptom of vascular disease manifesting itself as an erection problem. The guy really needs to see a cardiologist, especially because it's the same process as heart disease, just a different organ of the body showing that it's suffering from impaired blood flow."

But unless you and your wife have been living in a health news deprivation chamber for the past decade, you probably know that a growing number of experts believe that vitamin E could be a key to avoiding cardiovascular problems. What you may not know, however, is that vitamin E may also help you avoid erectile dysfunction.

The Virtues of Vitamin E

For many of us, just the thought of rubbing warm oil on that special someone gets the blood flowing. But it's the vitamin E found in things like almond and corn oil, nuts, even mayonnaise that gets some researchers all worked up.

Vitamin E may slow the rate at which blood thickens, and fatty goo called plaque sticks to the walls of your arteries, says Howard N. Hodis, M.D., director of the atherosclerosis research unit at the University of Southern California School of Medicine in Los Angeles.

"There are a lot of things that vitamin E does specifically," says Dr. Hodis. "It's an antioxidant. It can slow the rate of platelet aggregation and may therefore slow heart disease. It may even have direct, positive effects on arterial walls. But the bottom line is that it appears to help blood flow more smoothly."

Or at least that's the implication from the massive Health Professionals Follow-Up Study. Researchers followed 39,910 men for four years. Those men who had the highest vitamin E intake—primarily through supplements—had a 40 percent lower risk of coronary disease than the rest of the guys.

Would such an effect also allow blood to flow more smoothly to your penis, leading to firmer erections or helping you avoid erectile dysfunction altogether? Although more research needs to be done, the answer is probably yes. "You can quote me on this. Everything that you would think is good for your heart would be good for your penis. We just need more data," says Dr. Whitehead.

Even Dr. Hodis's research shows that those who took just 100 international units (IU) or more of vitamin E per day had less gooey plaque buildup in the arteries. Yet he is reluctant to recommend getting more than 30 IU, the recommended Daily Value of vitamin E. "Vitamin E is inexpensive and may be of great benefit if there's no downside to it," says Dr. Hodis. "But we need a few more years of data to feel comfortable recommending it as a supplement for heart disease. Those long-term studies are in the pipeline now. We'll know soon."

Meanwhile, more direct evidence linking vitamin E levels and erectile dysfunction continues to trickle in. Just like a coat of primer can keep an iron gate from rusting, antioxidants like vitamin E shield cells from harmful renegade molecules called free radicals. Suresh C. Sikka, Ph.D., associate professor of urology and director of the andrology clinic and research laboratories at the Tulane University School of Medicine in New Orleans, says that his studies show that vitamin E's antioxidant action may reduce free radical damage caused by diabetes, another common cause of erectile dysfunction. Dr. Sikka says his research shows that vitamin E thwarts the ability of free radicals to damage the smooth muscle cells in your penis that help you initiate and keep an erection.

But even while the benefits of vitamin E continue to build, most people don't get enough. And, ironically, some men may be getting less than ever—vitamin E, we mean. In a bid to cut back on their fat intake, health-conscious guys are using less vegetable oil and mayonnaise and, as a result, may be getting less vitamin E than recommended.

Potent Pills

You see them in the backs of men's magazines—ads for supplements that cleverly avoid making concrete claims about boosting your sexual prowess yet do a good job of, shall we say, raising your interest.

Unless you've tried them, it's hard to know whether they work. But judging from the ingredients on most of the labels, many contain enough herbs, vitamins, and minerals in one capsule to cover the gamut of male sexual complaints. A typical bottle reads like the contents of a sexual shaman's medicine bag: vitamin E, ginseng, ginkgo biloba, zinc, saw palmetto, and yohimbine, not to mention a hodgepodge of other ingredients, including amino acids and even caffeine. Now there's some evidence that vitamin E helps improve blood flow, and zinc is thought to aid fertility. But what about the rest of this stuff?

Originally used in China, ginseng is thought to be what's called an adaptogen, which means that it's supposed to help you better cope with stress, says William J. Keller, Ph.D., professor and chairman of the department of pharmaceutical sciences at Samford University in Birmingham, Alabama. "One possibility is that stress can cause a lack of sexual performance, so if you treat the stress, you may improve sexual performance," he says.

Ginseng also has been used successfully on conditions ranging from diabetes to clogged arteries, according to Varro E. Tyler, Ph.D., in his book The Honest Herbal.

Research shows that ginkgo biloba extract (GBE), made from the leaves of the ginkgo biloba tree, may help improve poor circulation, again one of the most common causes of erectile dysfunction, Dr. Keller says.

During one study 50 men diagnosed with erectile dysfunction received 240 milligrams of GBE daily for a period of nine months. Some of the men also received injections of the erection-boosting drug papaverine. The result: Erections in both groups improved, regardless of whether they received the extra injection. In an earlier study 30 patients who previously had not responded to papaverine injections regained potency after taking 60 milligrams of GBE daily for six months. Thirty others who participated in the study did not.

"Different compounds within ginkgo biloba facilitate blood flow," says Dr. Keller. "And as I understand it, these are supposed to increase circulation to the penis. Although more research needs to be done, it's another interesting possibility."

Saw palmetto has been found to help some cases of nonmalignant enlarged prostate, but there's less evidence that it increases sperm production or sexual vigor as some claim, according to Dr. Tyler.

The bark of an African tree, yohimbe, has been found by the Food and Drug Administration to enhance blood flow to the penis; but Dr. Keller says that you're more likely to experience benefits if you get the prescription version. It's called yohimbine hydrochloride.

Amino acid L-arginine has been reported to help boost libido and produce nitric oxide, which has been shown to help you keep an erection by holding blood in your penis. L-tyrosine, another amino acid that shows up in some formulas, is thought to combat depression, which can inhibit sexual desire, according to John Morgenthaler, Dan Joy, and Ward Dean in the book Better Sex through Chemistry.

But before you try any potency formula, you may want to check with your doctor. Many of the ingredients cause complications if you have an existing health condition. Yohimbine can interfere with blood pressure medications. GBE inhibits platelet aggregation, so be careful if you are taking anticoagulants. And if you have kidney stones, ask your doctor before taking zinc and other minerals.

Beating Stress and Fatigue

How to Energize Your Life

Unless you're an Arab sheik or enjoy waiting in line, the energy crisis of the 1970s isn't exactly what you'd call a fond memory.

But it wasn't all bad news. Not long after, American automakers began building more fuel-efficient cars like, well, the Chevy Chevette and the AMC Pacer.

The response to these innovations was overwhelming. People bought Toyotas and Hondas in record numbers. And only after the U.S. industry was on the verge of collapse did the guys in Detroit develop a few respectable fuel-efficient cars and perhaps their greatest achievement: crash-test dummies.

Don't wait until you're running like a four-cylinder rattle trap to deal with your personal energy crisis. A few simple, yet effective, nutritional changes can help banish stress and fatigue and increase your stamina to boot.

Defining Fatigue and Stress

Before you can take action, Jackson, you need to know what fatigue and stress are not. Let's start with fatigue. That incredible urge between 1:00 and 3:00 P.M. to wrap yourself in a down comforter and crawl under your desk? In the majority of cases, this is not fatigue but, rather, a natural decrease in alertness caused by your internal body clock—also known as your circadian rhythm. Jab yourself with a pencil or bang your head against your computer screen to stay awake if you must, but there's

probably something wrong with you if don't feel at least a little bit sleepy around this time.

"Post-lunch dip is an innate part of the biological rhythm that Americans are forced to fight. The rest of the world takes a siesta," says Michael H. Bonnet, Ph.D., director of the Sleep Laboratory at Dayton Veteran's Administration Hospital in Ohio.

Probably the best you can do to minimize the post-lunch slump—without resorting to caffeine—is to eat a light lunch devoid of alcohol, low in fat, and higher in protein and complex carbohydrates (like maybe tuna salad, which is high in protein, with romaine lettuce on a whole-grain roll, both of which are high in unrefined complex carbohydrates). And exercise if you have a chance, or at the very least, take a short, brisk walk, says Larry Christensen, Ph.D., chairman of the department of psychology at the University of South Alabama in Mobile.

Nor is fatigue defined by experts as the urge to sleep any other time of day. "If you can lie down, turn out the lights, and fall asleep, you're probably sleep-deprived. You're not getting enough sleep at night," Dr. Bonnet says. "When you're fatigued, you may feel tired, run-down, and listless. But if you turn off the lights, you won't be able to fall asleep either."

As for stress, put it this way: If fatigue is the glove, stress might be the hand. In other words, fatigue might be the result that others see, while stress is the real issue. Oftentimes, run-down people are actually stressed out over something physical—like injuries or a lack of proper nutrition—or over something psychological—like fear, anxiety, or anger. This may reflect an inextricable stress-nutrition connection. Stress can be an indirect cause of malnutrition or dietary deficiencies. What's more, your health nutrition-wise helps determine your body's ability to handle itself stress-

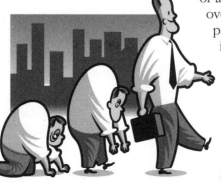

wise. For example, someone who suffers the physical stress of several multiple bone fractures in a car accident may require up to 30 percent more calories during the healing process alone.

The Energy Robbers

Ever seen an energetic wino? Been elbowed by a grump at the coffee machine? It should come as no surprise, then, that some guys with diets high in alcohol, caffeine, and sugar are more likely to suffer from fatigue.

A central nervous system depressant, alcohol can prevent you from getting restful sleep, which, of course, leads to sleep deprivation. Alcohol has been linked to depression, another common source of fatigue. Not only that, but booze also removes important vitamins from your system.

Caffeine can provide a 5-hour pick-me-up when you're suffering from fatigue—but only if you don't use it too often, says Dr. Bonnet. "Initially, people feel more energetic. But after drinking several cups of coffee a day for a week or two, they show signs of being overly aroused and actually report more fatigue. They have to drink more and more to get any effect," says Dr. Bonnet.

And although studies show that some depressed and fatigued guys crave sugar, the sweet stuff often makes them feel worse. "I've been with people who feel fatigued within a half-hour of eating something containing a lot of sugar. But then, look out," says Dr. Christensen. "Sugar desserts, snacks, whatever, can have a temporary lifting effect, but they prolong fatigue in many."

In the stress arena, energy robbers aren't usually what you put in your mouth but what

Melatonin: The Dream Drug?

Melatonin has been the subject of newsmagazine cover stories and best-selling books, touted by proponents as the elixir of immortality. But now that its 15 minutes of fame have passed, what remains is promising research that shows that you can change your sleep cycle by taking this natural neurotransmitter, says Dr. Michael H. Bonnet of the Sleep Laboratory at Dayton Veteran's Administration Hospital.

Found naturally in the brain, "melatonin sends the message to your body that it's time to shut down," says Dr. Bonnet. Unfortunately, as you get older your body produces less melatonin, making sleep more difficult. Supplementing melatonin apparently gives your body the same hit-the-sack message—even if it's not time. That means it could work really well, for example, for a guy changing from a night to a day job or who's suffering from jet lag.

Preliminary studies that indicated that melatonin may help ward off cancer, heart disease, high blood pressure, ulcers, migraines, Alzheimer's disease, and just about anything else you might develop have been tempered by millions who tried it in pill form and said they saw no benefit or reported such side effects as nightmares, stomach cramps, and low sex drive.

"We have yet to see a critical study that demonstrates that anything other than sleep is really affected by melatonin supplements," says Richard Spark, M.D., director of the Steroid Research Laboratory at Boston's Beth Israel Hospital and associate clinical professor of medicine at Harvard Medical School.

you put in your mind. Researchers have documented how physical stress affects the body nutritionally. They know that someone suffering from the physical stress of third-degree burns, for example, will need up to 40 percent more calories. What they don't know is exactly what nutritional toll psychological stress takes, since it varies greatly on an individual basis. This is the kind caused by downsizing, crime, family arguments, and love on the rocks. Preliminary research suggests that vitamin C might be promising, since the body seems to use more C when it's under stress. James Cason, Ph.D., retired professor of chemistry from the University of California, Berkeley, suggests vitamin C for stress protection based on studies on goats that show that a 150-pound goat will double the amount of vitamin C it makes when it's put under stress.

Shaken, Not Slurred

No one would confuse a saltshaker with a refueling station. But a growing number of researchers believe that the nationwide campaign to cut salt use has left millions sodium-deprived and, as a result, fatigued.

It's a controversial theory, and one that has drawn heat from the American Heart Association (AHA). For years, the AHA has suggested that we restrict salt use to lower our blood pressure in a bid to reduce our risk for a host of related diseases like heart disease and stroke. But Peter Rowe, M.D., associate professor of pediatrics and director of the diagnostic referral clinic of Johns Hopkins Children's Center in Baltimore, says that there's growing evidence that healthy sodium levels play a key role in keeping you energized.

"When you look at the older experiments in which sodium chloride intake was severely limited, all these studies describe a high frequency of malaise and fatigue occurring in research subjects," says Dr. Rowe.

Apparently, salt helps draw fluid into your bloodstream, which, in turn, keeps your blood volume up. Not enough salt, the theory goes, and your blood pressure can drop.

Such a drop probably isn't enough to slow you down, but guess what happens when you stand or sit all day at that desk of yours? Blood has a tendency to pool in your legs, decreasing the amount going to your heart. Combine the two, Dr. Rowe says, and your blood pressure may drop like a bad habit, leaving you light-headed and fatigued. Some folks even faint.

"It appears that the combination of inadequate amounts of salt and prolonged standing—waiting in line, showering, or quiet ambling, like when you shop—can bring this type of fatigue on," says Dr. Rowe. "Some athletes will get this after they finish a race or a sprint. For the most part, they're fine as long as they're running or moving during a sporting event. It's only when they are standing still in the cooldown period that they might feel light-headed or tired."

Adding salt and water to their diets should help reduce fatigue for those with mild symptoms, and these changes can be combined with medications for those with more severe symptoms—even for people with the mysterious, disabling condition known as chronic fatigue syndrome, says Dr. Rowe.

But what about all those public health messages to use less salt? "There has been a lot of well-intentioned hope in the advice about reducing sodium intake, but when researchers looked at 56 different salt-restriction studies, their conclusion was that the evidence that salt restriction lowers the blood pressures of normal individuals just isn't there," says Dr. Rowe.

But before you turn your saltshaker loose, check with your doctor. "If everything else seems okay, you and your physician together can make the judgment whether an increase in salt intake makes sense," says Dr. Rowe. The Daily Value for sodium is 2,400 milligrams.

Multiple Choice

Long considered little more than a nutritional insurance policy, there's evidence that the lowly multivitamin may be the Eveready Energizer bunny in capsule form. And yes, especially among those who seem to eat like life is one big lunch wagon.

Consider the results of a double-blind placebo controlled study—the strictest, most scientific kind—performed in England. Ninety-five middle managers were divided into two groups: those who received a multivitamin for eight weeks and those who took a fake pill. Researchers found that the folks who took the multivitamins (which also contained ginseng) and had the worst diets were more vigorous, less bewildered, and had better moods at the end of the study than those who swallowed the fake pills.

"The general conclusion…was that participants on a relatively poor diet benefited from taking dietary supplements in terms of moods and stress levels," the researchers wrote.

A much smaller, less-involved study looked at the nutrient intakes of depressed men and women but came to a similar conclusion. The study found that a substantial percentage (45 percent) of those who were depressed were getting less than the Daily Value of one or more nutrients.

And you don't have to be Perry Mason to see that the case for multivitamins is strengthened by a series of studies showing the effect of select nutrients on fatigue levels. Clinical studies, for example, have found that folks with low magnesium levels suffer from confusion, depression, anxiety, and insomnia—hallmarks of fatigue. Found in pumpkin seeds and sesame seeds and whole-grain cereals, magnesium has a Daily Value of 400 milligrams.

One of the same researchers who looked at the effects of low magnesium levels, James Penland, Ph.D., research psychologist at the U.S. Department of Agriculture–Agricultural Research Service Grand Forks Human Nutrition Research Center in North Dakota, raises similar concerns about selenium deficiencies. Dr. Penland found that guys who were fed a really low selenium diet (21 micrograms) for 15 weeks had more depression and confusion than guys chowing down on meals containing lots (180 micrograms) of this mineral. The Daily Value for sele-

nium is 70 micrograms. Be sure to consult your doctor first before supplementing your diet with more than 100 micrograms. Meats derived from muscle, as well as many cereals and dairy products, are really high in selenium.

Deficiencies in some B vitamins, including pantothenic acid (known as vitamin B_5) and vitamin B_{12}, for years have been linked to fatigue. In fact, a classic study shows that when male volunteers at the Iowa State Prison were fed a diet low in pantothenic acid, the convicts reported extreme fatigue, muscle weakness, sleepiness, and stomach distress, which, perhaps not so coincidentally, also happen to be popular stress symptoms. Researchers did not report, however, whether this affected their ability to produce license plates. Found in shiitake mushrooms, sunflower seeds, and eggs, pantothenic acid has a Daily Value of 10 milligrams.

The elderly are at great risk of developing B_{12} deficiency and often get B_{12} shots from their doctors to help them avoid the fatigue and other symptoms linked with deficiency. Although not completely understood, it's believed that as some people age, their digestive system loses some of its ability to digest and process vitamin B_{12} properly. A cup of Manhattan clam chowder has 132 percent of the B_{12} you need in a day, while pork and many ready-to-eat cereals are relatively good sources.

Vitamin C is also attracting some attention as a slump buster. In a study by the National Institute of Diabetes and Digestive and Kidney Diseases that looked at vitamin C blood and tissue levels, participants who got only 30 milligrams of vitamin C a day complained of feeling tired and irritable. Then there's the stress study we cited earlier about the goats, which suggests that you can keep stress from getting your goat by getting your vitamin C. The Daily Value for vitamin C is 60 milligrams, but even the institute has suggested that getting 200 milligrams is better. Guavas are jammed with vitamin C, as are sweet red peppers and, of course, orange juice.

Bolstering Your Immune System

Arm Yourself against Invaders

Nose hairs. Ugly, odd, and just one more part of the disease-fighting team that makes up your body's immune system, along with your skin, stomach lining, lymph glands, and a few thousand other apparently unrelated body parts.

You see, the immune system isn't really a "system" at all, at least not in the sense of a bunch of connected, interrelated parts like the nervous, digestive, or circulatory systems. It's more like the U.S. military complex: a disparate conglomerate of weaponry, bases, and uniquely trained soldiers all sharing just one thing—the goal of keeping your body from getting sick by blocking or killing unwelcome invaders.

Nose hairs, for example, trap bacteria and other particles that enter your nose as you breathe. And lymph glands manufacture and store white blood cells, which are among the most important players once an invading germ gets a foothold inside you.

The battle between your body and incoming germs rages on, day in and day out, with you having no clue of the details. All that is required of you is to constantly fuel your immune system to keep it strong and functioning.

Seeking Immunity

Medical researchers have known for decades that there is a strong link between good nutrition and the strength of your immune system. It's why infectious diseases kill most of the children who die in Third World

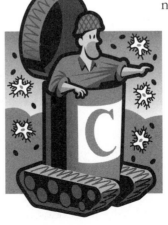

nations. But what is still being learned is exactly which nutrients are crucial to immunity. The medical community has discovered that several vitamins and minerals play a direct role in how well your body fights off germs and diseases. Here's what you need to maximize the many parts of your body's defense system.

Vitamin A. This is near the top of the list of vital nutrients for immunity. Vitamin A is essential to microbe-catching membranes in the mouth and respiratory passages. Doctors have identified a strong, direct link between vitamin A deficiency and the severity of respiratory diseases. Why? Without vitamin A, membranes in your mouth and throat might not repair correctly after infections, making them vulnerable to new infections.

Vitamin A also fortifies the top layer of skin, helping to prevent cracks through which invaders might enter. Getting the Daily Value of 5,000 international units should satisfy your immune system's needs.

Beta-carotene. Several studies have shown that beta-carotene bolsters immunity. In one study the number of T-helper cells in male volunteers jumped 30 percent after the men took 180 milligrams of beta-carotene daily for two weeks. (T-helper cells are important components of the immune system that are found in the bloodstream.) In another study at the University of Arizona in Tucson, men and women taking daily doses of 30 milligrams or more of beta-carotene for two months had noticeable improvements in immune response.

Vitamin B_6. Researchers at Tufts University School of Nutrition in Medford, Massachusetts, removed vitamin B_6 from the diets of healthy elderly people. The result was that immune response dropped substantially. When B_6 was reintroduced to the diets, immunity rebounded. But it took far more than the Daily Value of 2 milligrams to get back to previous immune power.

When participants took 50 milligrams daily, immunity was even better than before the study began.

Vitamin C. Who hasn't been taught that taking vitamin C helps fights colds? In reality, the vitamin bolsters your immune system to fight all diseases in a few ways. First and foremost, it is vital to the production of white blood cells, the foot soldiers of the immune system. White blood cells gather around cells in your body that have become infected, destroy them, then clean up the mess. Vitamin C also appears to stimulate white blood cells to function better. While an optimal level hasn't been determined, doctors believe that 500 milligrams daily is a good dosage to take care of immune system needs, along with all the other benefits that vitamin C provides.

Vitamin E. There has long been a positive link between this vitamin and immunity. In particular, supplementing with the vitamin appears to increase the levels of infection-fighting chemicals in the blood called interferon and interleukin. One study at Tufts University showed that supplementing with 800 milligrams daily of vitamin E increased interleukin-2 levels by 69 percent, while reducing the levels of a substance in the blood called prostaglandin that lowers white blood cell counts in your bloodstream.

Moreover, the antioxidant role of vitamin E helps your immune system. Research shows that when immune system cells kill and destroy viruses, bacteria, and other invaders, a by-product is free radicals. Vitamin E tames the free radicals. Experts believe that 400 international units of vitamin E per day is sufficient to bolster immunity.

Iron and zinc. When the body is exposed to an unexpected germ or particle, one of the things that happens is a sudden proliferation of immune cells. Both zinc and iron play a role in this. However, you don't need an abundance of either to get the job done—just the Daily Value of each. That's 18 milligrams for iron and 15 milligrams for zinc.

Magnesium. Some studies suggest that magnesium deficiency can cause the immune system to run amok, attack normal cells in the body, and trigger autoimmune diseases such as rheumatoid arthritis. Taking a magnesium supplement might be a good idea for men on water pills or high blood pressure drugs. Both make you lose the mineral, as does excessive alcohol intake. The rest of us can get by on the Daily Value of 400 milligrams.

One a Day Keeps Doc Away

For the committed vitamin gobbler, one of the core questions is whether to take a multivitamin or to supplement at higher levels vitamin by vitamin, pill by pill. When it comes to bolstering immunity, however, research suggests that a daily multivitamin just might do the trick.

In a yearlong study of 100 elderly Canadians, half the group received daily multivitamin/mineral supplements with extra vitamin E and beta-carotene. The other half got placebos—fake pills. At the end of the study, those on supplements had half as many colds, flus, and other infection-related illnesses as the group on placebos. And when they did get sick, those on supplements recovered in half the time.

Another study that tested the immune responses of people on multivitamins produced similar results. In this case, researchers used skin tests to measure the body's response to proteins taken from bacteria and fungi that cause some serious diseases, including tuberculosis and tetanus. After one year, those taking a multivitamin with minerals had a significantly more virile immune system than those taking placebos.

Looking Great

Make Your Appearance Healthy

An old-time Western explorer didn't look anything like Clint Eastwood, no matter how much he squinted. Living off dry rations all winter, he was woefully deficient in vitamins and minerals come spring. As a result, his skin was dry and rough, covered in reddish-blue spots. His swollen gums were bleeding, his lips and tongue inflamed. There were cracks on his lips and a flaky skin rash on parts of his body exposed to the sun. He was nothing to set Miss Kitty's heart aflutter.

All this says that vitamins and minerals are absolutely necessary for healthy skin and appearance. But all that's required to achieve this is getting the Daily Values, which, by now, you know are not that hard to get. The question is, can taking extra vitamins *improve* how you look?

Probably not. But, some vitamins and minerals—mostly those that are part of your body's antioxidant defense system—are being used to help skin problems heal better and, in some cases, prevent problems from occurring.

Sunshine Superman

The sun is responsible for the majority of changes that your skin undergoes as you age, according to Karen Burke, M.D., Ph.D., a dermatologist and dermatological surgeon in private practice in New York City. Ultraviolet radiation from the sun produces droves of free radicals at the same time it compromises your skin's antioxidant defenses. Prolonged exposure damages the elastic collagen fibers that make your skin resilient. When those fibers break down, wrinkles

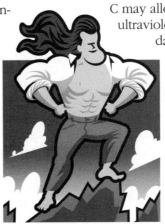

form. Sun damage also starts the process that can lead to skin cancer.

You can repair the ravages of the sun with tretinoin, a derivative of vitamin A, says Melvin L. Elson, M.D., medical director of the Dermatology Center in Nashville. The prescription topical medication Renova—which is tretinoin in a moisturizing base—has been approved by the Food and Drug Administration to treat fine lines and wrinkles and fade brown spots. It works by enhancing the production of collagen and forming thicker, moister epidermis, the top layer of your skin. The result is smoother skin.

Here are other ways to use vitamins to deflect the sun's harm.

Soothe with selenium. While all the antioxidant vitamins help protect the skin from sun damage, the mineral selenium appears to shine brightest. "If you have enough selenium, you won't get as many blistering sunburns," Dr. Burke says. "Because you get fewer sunburns, you have less aging of the skin and fewer skin cancers." Depending on the soil levels of selenium where you live, Dr. Burke recommends 50 to 200 micrograms of selenium in the more biologically available form, l-selenomethionine. Doses above this amount should only be taken under medical supervision. Good food sources of selenium include grains (tabbouleh is high on Dr. Burke's list) or saltwater fish, especially salmon.

Apply C at the sea. Topical vitamin C may allow the skin to withstand more ultraviolet exposure without getting as damaged, says Thomas N. Helm, M.D., assistant clinical professor of dermatology at the State University of New York at Buffalo School of Medicine and Biomedical Sciences. In studies at Duke University Medical Center, skin pretreated with vitamin C had less severe sunburns than untreated skin.

Heal burns with E. If you do get a sunburn, "take 400

international units (IU) of vitamin E every 4 hours starting immediately after the burn and continuing for one or two days," suggests Dr. Burke. "The d-alpha-tocopherol form is best." (You may want to check with your doctor first, especially if you are on certain blood-thinning medications).

Battle cancer with A. Vitamin A and vitamin A derivatives like tretinoin may also play an important role in preventing skin cancer. In one study, people with a high risk for skin cancer because of earlier sun damage were given 25,000 IU of vitamin A each day. "The people who got vitamin A developed fewer squamous cell cancers than those who didn't get vitamin A," says Norman Levine, M.D., chief of dermatology at the University of Arizona Health Sciences Center in Tucson. "The dosage we used was fairly high, but our patients didn't get many reactions. Still, at this level it is no longer a vitamin; it is a drug." Dosages above 15,000 IU should only be taken under medical supervision.

Healing the Skin

Oral and topical vitamins can also help restore your skin to normal if it has been injured or if you suffer from psoriasis. "If I had a serious burn or surgery, I would carefully watch my nutrition intake and take a multivitamin with minerals," says Dr. Helm. "You want to cover the whole spectrum."

Dr. Burke suggests taking 400 IU of vitamin E. "It helps wound healing and is excellent for preventing raised scars or keloids. Just don't take it right before surgery, since it is a mild anticoagulant."

A synthetic form of prescription topical vitamin D, called calcipotriene (Dovonex), has proven effective in reducing plaques, red, itchy, scaly raised patches on knees and elbows, which are the hallmarks of psoriasis. "If we use it on 100 patients, ⁴⁄₅ of them show some improvement. For 15 percent, it is almost a home run hit," says Dr. Helm. For severe psoriasis, prescription etretinate (Tegison), a superpotent

form of vitamin A, is given orally and only under a doctor's strict supervision.

The Happy Head

Want to use vitamins to achieve healthy hair and a happy smile? Here's what works.

Nourish the living. The hair you see is dead, so fancy vitamins in shampoos aren't going to help any. You need to nourish the living follicle inside your skin. "I recommend 1,000 milligrams of L-cysteine, an essential amino acid, plus 3,000 milligrams of vitamin C and 400 IU of vitamin E," says Dr. Burke. "I give this to anyone with hair problems. And a B-complex vitamin can't hurt either." One caution: Taking more than 1,200 milligrams of vitamin C may cause diarrhea in some people. Check with your doctor before supplementing at high levels.

Build a firm foundation. By now, your teeth have finished forming, But the bone supporting your teeth is continually broken down and rebuilt. It needs a continual supply of calcium and vitamin D to stay strong. Too little of these nutrients, and the bone supporting your teeth could weaken, says Heidi K. Hausauer, D.D.S., spokesperson for the Academy of General Dentistry and assistant clinical professor at the University of the Pacific Dental School's department of operative dentistry in San Francisco. In extreme cases you could even lose some teeth. In the healthy, periodontal disease–free person the Daily Value of calcium is enough. Some people with osteoporosis may need more, says Dr. Hausauer.

Attack gum disease with C. "A vitamin C deficiency alone does not cause gingivitis," says Dr. Hausauer. "You have to have a local irritant like plaque or tartar to get it. But people with a vitamin C deficiency have worse symptoms, such as bone loss, bleeding gums, and tooth loosening and loss." So prevent gum disease two ways: through smart mouth maintenance (brushing, flossing, and regular professional dental visits) and by getting enough vitamin C in your diet. Make sure that you get at least the Daily Value of vitamin C.

Building Muscle

Make the Most of What You Have

From drinking raw eggs à la Rocky to gulping pills made out of powdered bull testicles, few pursuits have challenged the imagination—or the palette—as the quest to build muscle.

Unfortunately, much of this effort—Herculean as it may seem—is nothing more than a giant-size con job. Many so-called muscle-building supplements, if based on any science at all, routinely cite studies that only hint at possible muscle growth in animals. And that's great news—if you're an underweight laboratory rat or monkey.

Other manufacturers actually boast about their products with little more than data showing effects of certain nutrients on burn victims or folks who have been hospitalized. This could also be encouraging, especially if you're routinely carried into the gym on a stretcher.

But perhaps worst of all: Many marketing campaigns play on the shortcut-to-muscle mentality that drives some weight lifters to use dangerous anabolic steroids.

But you don't have to die pencil-necked and penniless. There's solid evidence that supplementing your diet with several nutrients, while resistance-training, can help you build muscle.

The Muscles of Your Dreams

In the movie Field of Dreams, Kevin Costner's character is haunted by a voice that says, "If you build it, he will come." Decent movie, great concept—for weight lifters, not Iowa farmers.

When you're trying to build muscle, repeat this to yourself (without moving your lips, of course): "If I tear them down, my muscles will grow."

Here's why: Like a tightly woven rope, your muscles are composed of fibers—tiny, water-saturated strands ranging in size from a few millimeters to those running the length of your thigh, your body's longest. Roughly divided into fast-twitch and slow-twitch fibers, each has a specific purpose. Fast-twitch muscle fibers help you sprint to victory. Slow-twitch muscle fibers provide the aerobic endurance in your legs to keep you chugging during a weekend 10-K.

Now, we all know someone who is blessed (or cursed, depending on how you look at it) with more or less of both. Surrounded by women, Mr. Fast Twitch seems to only glance at a weight and his biceps swell. And Mr. Slow Twitch? He's the guy in the corner without a date, impersonating a string bean. "You there, are those your calves—or are you walking on stilts?"

Bad as it may seem, all is not lost for Mr. Slow Twitch or his scrawny brethren. With the right training, nutrients, and rest, they can also develop more muscle—safely and naturally. "It's hard to compensate for less-than-optimal genetics," says Kathy K. Grunewald, Ph.D., professor in the department of foods and nutrition at Kansas State University in Manhattan and the author of a study that investigated commercially marketed body-building supplements. "But you can maximize the expression of your genetics with the right eating habits, training program, and rest."

Let's say that you don't lift weights very often. In fact,

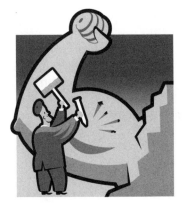

let's say that you'd rather listen to testimonials for a psychic hotline than lift weights. But whether you're working out or watching cable TV around-the-clock, your muscle cells break down every 7 to 15 days.

Weight training actually forces those cells to break down and rebuild faster—even in as little as 48 hours. And with the right training program, good nutrition, and rest, muscle growth follows. Size. Mass. You may not be able to do anything about your genetics, but you can train your slow-twitch muscles to perform like fast-twitch ones—and vice versa. You'll definitely grow stronger while looking and feeling better.

The Power of Protein

The typical American male easily gets the Daily Value of protein in his diet. And for the longest time, some nutrition experts said that you didn't need any more than that—regardless of your exercise program.

But research shows that eating an extra 60 to 70 grams of high-quality protein a day above and beyond the Daily Value (50 grams), combined with proper rest and weight training, will enhance muscle building. That's about two extra cans of tuna a day.

Simply put, your digestive system breaks down that protein into amino acids, which are then synthesized by your body and delivered through your blood to your muscles. If your muscles have been broken down with weight training, they tap the amino acids to rebuild, creating new contractile protein, also known as muscle tissue.

And there are plenty of ways to get more protein in your diet. "It could be soy or whey protein if you don't want to eat meat. Or casein, which is the protein found in milk," says Craig Cisar, Ph.D., professor of exercise physiology in the department of human performance at San Jose State University in California. In fact, many of the protein supplements on sale at your local

health food store are made from casein. You can also combine incomplete proteins to make complete proteins, the perennial example being eating beans and rice.

Or you can buy some inexpensive nonfat dry milk and add it to your next low-fat shake to create a super drink that, combined with strength training, can help pack on muscular pounds.

"That would cost far less than what you would pay for some protein in a can," Dr. Cisar says. Or try any other low-fat animal protein like chicken or egg whites. And keep your fat intake between 20 and 25 percent of your daily calories.

Consider Creatine

In some nutritional research circles, they call Peter Lemon, Ph.D., "Mr. Protein." Not because he eats a lot of protein, but as the director of the Applied Physiology Research Laboratory at Kent State University in Kent, Ohio, his research has made a convincing case that weight lifters and bodybuilders need more protein.

But soon he may be better known for his creatine research. During a creatine study in which he was both a participant and an author, Dr. Lemon was surprised to discover that his shirts got tighter in all the right places—and it wasn't because he left them in the dryer too long.

"It was a noticeable change," says Dr. Lemon. "When we started this study, we really didn't know the kind of effect we were going to get. But it was that big. You could tell."

In what's called a double-blind, placebo-controlled, crossover study, men were divided into two groups: those who were given creatine and didn't know it and those who were given a fake substance and didn't know it. The interesting part is that it wasn't long before some guys were pretty sure who was taking what.

"We didn't document this for our study

because we were just looking at the effects of creatine on one exercise. But the guys were saying that they could do more weight, more reps. They just felt stronger during their free weight workouts, myself included," says Dr. Lemon.

When it finally came time to do some measuring for the actual study, the results were just as impressive. After taking a start-up "loading" dose of 20 grams of creatine a day, the guys were able to generate 8 to 10 percent more force in a modified calf raise. Their calves, on average, increased in size by 3.4 percent.

And, oh yeah—some guys gained as much as 6 pounds after just one week of weight training! "It was a phenomenal increase in performance and a dramatic weight gain," says Dr. Lemon.

And it's not the only study to document increased power and weight gains in men who take creatine. In bench press studies, guys boosted both their one-rep max and reps with 70 percent of their max—even when doing five sets. Sprinters bested their 300- and 1,000-meter times. Cyclists pedaled faster for short distances. And in at least seven studies, all the guys using creatine gained weight—from about 2 pounds to 4 pounds.

"One of our graduate students did the same kind of study here with baseball players, and in one week they gained nearly 5 pounds," says Melvin Williams, Ph.D., professor of exercise science at Old Dominion University in Norfolk, Virginia. "After that we put them on a maintenance dose for two weeks down to 5 to 10 grams per day, and they maintained the weight gain. And then they went off creatine supplements for another week and still maintained it."

Add Some Antioxidants

Normally, you wouldn't talk about smoking, smog, and muscle building in the same breath. But when it comes to generating free radicals—those misguided molecules that bounce around your body damaging tissues—heavy weight training may be in the same league. That's because the sudden, dramatic increase of oxygen needed to fuel your weight training generates lots of free radicals.

But from a muscle building standpoint, probably the worst thing about free radicals is that they may play a role in cutting short your marathon runs (or cycling): in other words, fatigue. At least that was the conclusion of studies conducted at the Baylor College of Medicine, according to Chandan K. Sen, Ph.D., a research biochemist in the department of molecular and cell biology at the University of California, Berkeley.

"These studies showed clearly the role of free radicals in fatigue and stirred up much interest in the possible role of antioxidants and muscle performance," Dr. Sen says.

Fortunately, your body does have some built-in antioxidant defenses. The bad news is that they often can't get the job done on their own and, in fact, seem less capable of coping with the problem as the years go by.

"Several studies have shown that with aging, you may start losing some of your antioxidant defense ability—your antioxidant defense status literally downshifts," says Dr. Sen.

So how does this creatine work? More research needs to be done, of course, but this much we know. Creatine is found naturally in your muscles and in almost all animal meat: beef, pork, chicken, turkey, fish, and others. Un-

But simply popping some vitamin E, famous for its antioxidant power, might not be enough to protect your from those ravaging free radicals. In fact, some free radicals are so tough that they can attack and overwhelm your antioxidants, creating a damaging buildup of impotent antioxidant derivatives that may cause muscle damage.

So how do you fight back? "Studies have shown that if you want to recycle or rejuvenate vitamin E in your muscle, you need vitamin C and a critically important amino acid trio called glutathione that is synthesized in the muscle," Dr. Sen says.

Although the Daily Value for vitamin E is 30 international units (IU), some experts suggest taking 200 to 400 IU to see any effect. If you are considering taking amounts above 600 IU, discuss it with your doctor first.

The Daily Value for vitamin C is 60 milligrams, the amount found in a small orange, but many people take much more. Side effects, though unusual, may include diarrhea or kidney stones.

Glutathione is produced in the body if three amino acids are present, including cysteine, which can be obtained from both meat and plant sources. If you exercise or lead an active lifestyle, muscle increases its capacity to make glutathione.

The reverse is also true. Muscle that is not regularly exercised loses this capability, according to Dr. Sen.

phosphocreatine—a ready fuel for high-intensity exercise like weight training. On the other hand, heavy lifting apparently depletes your muscles' creatine phosphate stores quickly—unless, it seems, they've been saturated with extra creatine. Once your muscles reach the saturation point, research shows that you're able to work out harder with more weight—a prime builder of muscle tissue over time. And that's a key point because it's likely that much of the muscle size and weight gained in a week when you're using creatine is water being drawn into your muscle fibers. But it's probably only a matter of time before those strength gains and more intense training sessions produce even more muscle, says Dr. Lemon.

It appears that once you reach your saturation point, you may not need to continue taking 20 grams; you can cut back to 5 to 6 grams a day after your first week, says Dr. Lemon. In fact, after the initial loading , it may even be possible to keep those creatine levels topped off without any supplementation as long as you're eating a lot of meat and fish, foods that contain high levels of creatine, Dr. Lemon says.

"It's like if you're training as hard as you can and I somehow give you a magic potion that enables you to train 10 percent harder. It almost sounds too good to be true," says Dr. Lemon. "I think we're going to be looking at this stuff for a while." However, a word of caution is necessary because, as yet, long-term studies with these creatine dosages have not been completed. Although no adverse side effects of creatine supplementation have been observed, it may be that prolonged usage could eventually cause problems.

fortunately, you'd need to eat about 10 pounds of meat to get the same amount that the guys used as a loading dose in the study: 20 grams.

After you eat creatine, studies show, it's stored in your muscles as what's called

Losing Weight

Eat Your Way to a Slender Frame

Remember crash diets? They were fine if you were a crash-test dummy. But for flesh-and-blood men, they didn't work.

The pattern went like this: You'd eat nothing but the occasional grapefruit or dollop of cottage cheese. You'd walk around for a few days feeling weak, deprived, and crabby. Then you'd quit the diet in frustration and dive into a three-day pizza and ice cream binge. In the long run, you didn't lose weight…you lost friends.

Even if you had the willpower to stick to a deprivation diet long enough to lose a few pounds, you'd be making a big mistake. Your bodily systems will not function without the nutrients that come with regular, sensible eating, nutrition experts say. This leads us to a weight-loss rule you'll love: Make sure that you get enough to eat.

Very low calorie diets are out—way out. Modern man has evolved to a more satisfying way of eating to lose or maintain weight. "Men need more calories than women, in general, to get all the nutrients they need. A man must make sure that he consumes enough while on a weight-loss program," says Gail Frank, R.D., Dr. P.H., professor of nutrition at California State University, Long Beach, and nutritional epidemiologist. So eating moderately, in a nutritionally balanced way, is the key to successful weight loss, she says. Besides, if you eat enough food to prevent feeling deprived, it will be easier to keep up your healthier eating habits over the long haul.

Here are some tips to help you lose the pounds you

want without losing vital nutrients.

Make every calorie count. Vitamins and minerals do not help you lose weight faster, but they are important in your weight-loss program. "Vitamins and minerals help in the metabolism of fat, carbohydrate, and protein. If you aren't getting enough of these nutrients because of your weight-loss plan, you run the very real risk of interfering with these functions," says Dr. Frank. Many vitamins and minerals help each other get absorbed better, too. So to make every calorie count, don't just fill your gut—choose foods that are packed with these nutrients.

Do the math. So how many calories do you have to consume in order to get enough nutrients and still lose weight? There's a formula that you can use to determine the lowest number of calories you should allow, says Leslie Bonci, R.D., nutritionist at the University of Pittsburgh Medical Center and dietitian for the NFL's Pittsburgh Steelers and University of Pittsburgh athletics department. "Men should multiply their weight in pounds by 11," she says. That means that a 180-pound man should consume at least 1,980 calories a day. You can usually take in about 200 calories above this number and still lose weight, says Bonci, who also is a spokesperson for the American Dietetic Association (ADA). Height, activity level, and various health conditions also play a factor, so if you are looking for an exact caloric plan, it's best to be evaluated by a dietitian.

Diversify your assets. Make variety your dietary motto. "There are so many low-fat and fat-free choices of vegetables, fruits, and grains available in today's supermarkets, it's easier than ever to keep your vitamin and mineral sources interesting and diverse," says Bonci. If getting variety into your regular meals is hard for you to arrange, eat lots of different fruits and vegetables as snacks throughout

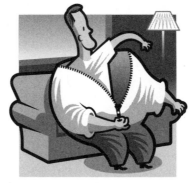

the day. Then you can eat smaller portions of your usual fare at mealtime.

Ponder a multi-pill. If you're restricting the calories you consume to lose weight, you may want to consider taking a multivitamin/mineral supplement, but only as an addition to a nutritious diet. "They are called supplements and not substitutes for a reason. Relying on supplements to take care of your micronutrient needs is like putting an adhesive bandage on a gaping wound," says Bonci. It won't replace eating the complex arrangements of nutrients found in healthy foods. A supplement can, however, act as nutritional insurance in case you accidentally fall short of any of your essential nutrients from one day to the next.

Accelerate the process. It all seems like a frustrating catch-22: You want to lose weight, but to prevent wrecking your body in the process you have to keep up your nutrient consumption, which means eating. This means more calories, which get stored as body fat if they aren't burned up.

If you want to accelerate the weight-loss process, then shave off those excess calories by stepping up your physical activity. "You can achieve your weight-loss goals and nutritional goals at the same time and obtain other health benefits by incorporating exercise into your moderate-calorie weight-management plan," says Dr. Frank. Exercising will increase the amount of calories your body burns throughout the day, not just when you are working out. A very low calorie diet won't do that for you.

Contrary to one popular myth, exercise has no effect on vitamin or mineral absorption in men. "Exercise does affect how the

No Substitute for Good Eating

Processed nonfat and low-fat snack foods might help you shave some fat out of your diet. But the trouble is that most of these products contain refined carbohydrates—basically sugar—and they offer zip for vitamins or minerals. Check the label. Steer clear of snacks low in fat but having less than 10 percent of Daily Values for vitamins and minerals or you will be eating truly empty calories, says Dr. Gail Frank of California State University, Long Beach. Some better choices include a banana, an orange, a bagel with apple butter, carrot sticks with salsa, or some other naturally low-fat food that provides nutrients along with its calories.

"Fat-soluble vitamins are forfeited when a person restricts all dietary fat for these fat-substitute products," says Anne Dubner, R.D., a dietitian in Houston who has worked with the NFL's Houston Oilers and is a spokesperson for the American Dietetic Association. Vitamins A, D, E, and K all need a little fat in order to be absorbed by the body. "I tell my patients to aim for 20 percent of total calories from fat because, that way, if they underestimate the fat in foods or cheat on this plan a little, they will still be able to lose weight and maintain proper fat-soluble vitamin absorption," she says.

Don't assume that a multivitamin/mineral supplement will help offset the excessive use of processed snack foods. A pill could never replicate the vast combinations of known and unknown nutrients locked inside fruits, vegetables, whole grains, and other naturally low-fat foods, says Dr. Frank.

body uses fat, protein, and carbohydrate; but it does not affect the body's use of vitamins and minerals," says the ADA's Anne Dubner.

Eating a Vegetarian Diet

Be a B$_{12}$ Booster

Okay, we're going to play a little visualization game. Picture a typical serving plate at a typical American restaurant. What does it look like? Big slab of meat. A heaping spoonful of potatoes, rice, or noodles. And over in the corner, a small pile of vegetables that you could count individually without even having to use your toes. Now, take away the meat. What do you fill the plate with?

Vegetarians face that choice daily. Whatever their personal reasons for eschewing, as opposed to chewing, meat, vegetarians gain a distinct advantage over their meat-eating brethren in getting the upper levels of the recommended servings of fruit and vegetables each day. Their diets also are likely to be lower in saturated fats and higher in vitamins, minerals, and fiber, calorie per calorie.

But when you take away the meat, you may be taking away something else, something very important for men: vitamin B$_{12}$. Also called cobalamin, this nutrient is vital to the production of myelin, which insulates nerve fibers and helps keep electrical impulses moving through the body.

Vitamin B$_{12}$ is also important in the production of red blood cells. In its natural form, vitamin B$_{12}$ is found exclusively in animal products, such as red meat, dairy products, fish, and eggs. The Daily Value for vitamin B$_{12}$ is only 6 micrograms, but this scant amount is essential.

"Long-term deficiencies in B$_{12}$ can result in irreversible nerve damage. This can be a concern, depending on the type of vegetarian diet a person subscribes to," says Anne Dubner of the American Dietetic Association (ADA).

Getting Enough

Vegetarian diets that include animal products, but not meat, can generally offer enough vitamin B$_{12}$ to ward off deficiency, says Dubner, who also has served as a dietitian for the NFL's Houston Oilers. Lacto vegetarians (those who eat dairy products like cheeses and milk) and lacto-ovo vegetarians (those who eat dairy products and eggs), for example, can usually get plenty of B$_{12}$ without too much effort by incorporating dairy products and fortified cereals and breads into their diets. Vegetarians who also eat seafood have it even easier, since foods such as clams, tuna, and salmon are good sources of B$_{12}$.

Vegans, who do not eat any animal-based foods whatsoever, are the vegetarians who need to really think hard about where they can get their B$_{12}$. "True vegans have to supplement their vitamin B$_{12}$ supply somehow; there's no way around it," Dubner says. "Luckily, there are simple ways to do this."

For starters, vegetarians who are concerned about their B$_{12}$ consumption should eat breakfast cereals and breads that are fortified with vitamin B$_{12}$, Dubner says. Use the B$_{12}$ information on the nutrition label to help you select these products. A daily multivitamin/mineral supplement also can provide your daily supply of the essential vitamin.

Because excessive amounts of B$_{12}$ are excreted in the urine, supplementing this vitamin is considered extremely safe, even in large doses.

You may have heard about vitamin-B$_{12}$ shots for senior citizens whose bodies no longer properly absorb the nutrient. "That's really unnecessary for a vegetarian because there

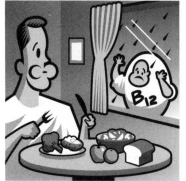

are so many easier ways to get adequate amounts of vitamin B$_{12}$," Dubner says.

Other Needs

Here are some other pointers that vegetarians should keep in mind.

Iron out your problems. Vegetarians can sometimes shortchange themselves when it comes to iron. That's because the heme iron found in meat is easily absorbed by the body, while the nonheme iron found in plant foods is less absorbable. Because too much iron in the diet has been linked to heart disease in men, supplementation is not generally recommended. So what's a guy to do?

"Vegetarians can easily make up for the amount of readily absorbable iron found in meat by consuming vitamin C and iron together," says Leslie Bonci of the University of Pittsburgh Medical Center and the NFL's Pittsburgh Steelers. Vitamin C consumed with iron increases the mineral's absorption. Plant foods that contain a good supply of iron include dark green, leafy vegetables (such as spinach), hot breakfast cereals (such as Cream of Wheat), dried beans, dried fruit, and soybean products. When you eat these foods, increase their effectiveness by also having vitamin C–rich foods, such as a glass of orange juice, red bell pepper slices, or maybe some tomato wedges.

Bone up. By not eating meat, vegetarians may protect their bones from future fractures and deformities. Several studies have shown that excessive consumption of animal protein is linked to an increased calcium loss through the urine. This may increase a person's risk of developing osteoporosis, a debilitating bone-thinning disease.

The Pseudo Solution

If you're like most men, you just can't go cold turkey when it comes to meat. But if you're tempted by the health benefits of vegetarianism, you don't have to go whole hog. It may actually be to your advantage to cut back rather than cut out meat. Join the ranks of the pseudo-vegetarians.

Instead of giving up all meat all the time, do the next best thing and give up all meat (that is, beef, pork, and poultry) most of the time. "You'll get all the B$_{12}$ and iron you'll need, without feeling deprived of the taste of meat," says Anne Dubner of the American Dietetic Association.

Cut down your meat consumption to one 3-ounce portion (about the size of a deck of playing cards) a day. Save it for the meal where it would give you the most satisfaction, Dubner recommends. Fill the rest of your meals and snacks with other types of foods, such as whole grains, fruits, and vegetables. After a few weeks, you may even want to cut back to having meat only a few days a week, says Dubner.

"One way to make sure that you stick with a pseudo-vegetarian program is to indulge yourself with the freshest or most flavorful varieties of produce and grains," Dubner says. "Spoil yourself with the meat alternatives." Use part of the money that you'd normally spend on several large cuts of lesser-quality meat on one good 3-ounce cut, then spend the rest on the best quality of fruits and vegetables you can find, Dubner recommends.

Since this has not been found to be the case with vegetable-protein sources, vegetarians may actually have a lower risk for osteoporosis than meat-eaters. "Lacto vegetarians have been shown to have good bone density," Bonci says.

Strategies for Vegetable-Haters

11 Ways to Get What You Need

You know that you're supposed to eat three to five servings of vegetables a day. You know that vegetables are loaded with disease-fighting and health-promoting vitamins and minerals. You know that they contain other mysterious nutrients that scientists haven't even pinpointed yet. And you know that you can't get the same nutritional boost from some pill.

There's just one problem: You hate vegetables.

"Ask yourself, 'What do I hate about vegetables?' If it's the way you were served them as a kid, that can be changed," says Anne Dubner of the American Dietetic Association (ADA).

The Energizing Eleven

Let's be honest: There are some vegetables that you're just not going to eat, regardless of how they're prepared. That's fine. But there are a lot of others that may surprise you. All it takes is a dash of creativity and an open mind.

Here are 11 (call it a vegetable-hater's dozen) expert tips you can use to painlessly—perhaps even deliciously—increase the number and variety of vegetables in your daily diet.

Eat 'em raw. Cooking can cause vegetables to lose some of their nutrients. If you aren't getting many vegetables to begin with, stick to uncooked ones to get the maximum nutritional benefits. "Some people just can't stand the sight, smell, texture, or taste of cooked spinach. But they will gladly eat

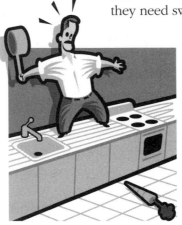

a spinach salad," Dubner says. Raw vegetables tend to be brighter, fresher-smelling, and crispier than ones that have been cooked, especially in boiling water. Raw vegetables can often taste more lively, too. "If all you've ever had are mushy, overcooked vegetables, try the raw versions and you won't believe how much better they taste," Dubner says.

Flash 'em. When cooking vegetables in water, let the pot reach a rolling boil first. Then drop in the vegetables, count to 10, and drain them. This method of cooking, called flash-boiling, retains more vitamins in vegetables than longer methods of cooking, says Dubner. Other cooking methods that limit nutrient loss are steaming, stir-frying, and microwaving.

Sneak 'em in. "Try adding vegetables to recipes that have so much stuff going on, you won't notice that anything has been added," says Leslie Bonci of the University of Pittsburgh Medical Center and the NFL's Pittsburgh Steelers. Bulk up your favorite casserole, soup, lasagna, or chili with chopped or shredded vegetables. The added ingredients will take on the flavorings of the dish, making them painlessly disappear from your plate.

Add spice. If you think that plain vegetables taste boring, spice them with your favorite seasonings, herb, hot sauce, or soy sauce. Dubner recommends throwing dill on steamed carrots, or oregano on flash-boiled green beans. You also can glaze your vegetables with a small amount of honey or sugar if they need sweetening.

Enjoy your salad days. "A lot of people who hate vegetables will still eat salads," Dubner says. "If you can agree to at least eat some salad with your meals, you're doing a lot of good." Salads can be a great diet-enhancing tool. Salads made from a wide assortment of produce give you variety as well as nutrients, says Dubner. Every cup of salad equals one serving of vegetables, as long as it's not the cheapo kind—you know, a quarter head of iceberg lettuce thrown in a bowl with some dressing.

If you don't mind eating salads but can't seem to find the time or patience to prepare your own, supermarket salad bars take away the hassle of preparation, says Dubner. Buy ready-to-eat packages of greens so that you don't have to wash and chop them at home. When you eat out, order a salad whenever it comes with your entrée, and consider ordering one if it doesn't come with your meal. And yes, that includes fast-food restaurants, too. A side salad instead of a side order of fries can make a huge nutritional difference.

Be a big dipper. Pass on the chips and grab hold of some crisp vegetables when you crack open the onion dip, cheese spread, salsa, or some other enticing concoction. Have a bag of washed and cut vegetables ready in the refrigerator for when the mood hits you. Sugar snap peas, carrot sticks, and bell pepper wedges have excellent dip-scooping abilities. When the cupboard is bare, salad dressing makes a good veggie dip in a pinch, says Dubner.

Be extravagant. Some rich accompaniments can be used sparingly to make vegetables more appealing. "It's better to have some fat and get the vegetables in than it is to forfeit the produce all together," says Bonci. Try adding a bit of cheese or creamy sauce to your vegetables. If you are counting calories and fat for health or weight-loss reasons, use low-fat cheeses or condiments. Or consider having smaller portions or low-fat varieties of meats or desserts in order to allow yourself a more satisfying vegetable dish, says Bonci.

Batter up. Mild-tasting vegetables, such as zucchini, mushrooms, and squashes, can be coated with light or nonfat mayonnaise and bread crumbs, then baked in the oven to make them more palatable, says Bonci.

The Big Chill

Frozen and canned vegetables are equally convenient but are not always equally nutritious. "Frozen vegetables are flash-frozen not long after they are ripe so that the nutritional value stays quite high, naturally. Nothing is depleted from them," says Leslie Bonci of the University of Pittsburgh Medical Center and the NFL's Pittsburgh Steelers. However, when vegetables are canned, the B-vitamin levels drop during heating. That's because B vitamins aren't heat-stable.

"Of course, canned vegetables are better than none," says Bonci. So, if nothing else is available, grab a can opener.

Get juiced. Drinking a vegetable beverage, such as V-8 or carrot juice, is one way to get the vitamins and minerals of vegetables, although you lose out on the fiber, Dubner says. If you are eating whole-grain foods and fresh fruit, this shouldn't be a huge concern.

Get yelled at. "When you go shopping, look for the produce that has eye-catching color. Let the vegetables scream at you in the aisle," Dubner says. Bright colors are usually signs that the vegetables are rich in vitamins—just look at tomatoes, bell peppers, and carrots. Choose romaine lettuce over iceberg if you aren't buying a lot of produce. The washed-out color of iceberg lettuce is a hint that it contains few nutrients, Dubner says. Other vegetables, such as cucumbers and celery, have pale inside flesh that show that they are low in nutritional value.

When all else fails, eat fruit. Until you have gotten into the swing of eating vegetables, pad your diet with the other star of the produce aisle. "Fruit will provide most of the same vitamins and minerals. So if you like more of them, count some fruit as part of your three to five servings of vegetables each day," says Bonci.

Boosting Your Brainpower

Win the Battle for Your Heart and Mind

It doesn't matter whether you're Einstein or Ernest (the Jim Varney character who starred in such film classics as Ernest Scared Stupid and Ernest Goes to Camp). Theoretically, our brains all work pretty much the same way. That 3- to 4-pound chunk of gray matter nestled comfortably in your skull is laced with 100 billion brain cells called neurons. Featuring rootlike growths called axons and dendrites that loosely resemble the playoff pairings on the road to the Final Four, these neurons stretch toward one another. Close as they might get, however, your axons and dendrites are like most of the 64 teams in the National Collegiate Athletic Association basketball tournament each year—they never quite make it all the way.

But your neurons aren't supposed to connect. It's up to neurotransmitters such as dopamine, norepinephrine, serotonin, and acetylcholine to chemically bridge those tiny synaptic gaps. Once in place, however, your memories, thoughts, and ideas flow from axons and dendrites on one side of your brain to the other—all in less time than it takes to throw down a monster dunk at the end of a fast break.

Meanwhile, your heart, arteries, and blood vessels perform the less glamorous task of pumping blood to your brain, providing the oxygen and nutrients needed to create neurotransmitters and nourish brain cells. In fact, your brain consumes nearly 20 percent of the oxygen your body brings in.

You don't have to be Einstein to figure out what happens if fatty plaque builds on the walls of those vessels and arteries and alters the flow of blood. If the clog is bad enough, you could have a stroke and die. And if it's merely slowed? That might help explain Ernest. Although more research needs to be done, there's evidence that clogged arteries may contribute to seriously fuzzy thinking.

Go with the Flow

Researchers who analyzed mental performance tests given during the famed Framingham Heart Study found a link between increasing levels of high blood pressure and decreased mental acuity. It seems that the higher the blood pressure among the volunteers—a hallmark of cardiovascular disease—the lower they scored on memory and attention tests.

"Probably the hardest mental hits from high blood pressure are going to be in memory, but there's some degradation of cognitive function in general," says Merrill F. Elias, Ph.D., professor of psychology at the University of Maine in Orono and lead investigator on the study.

A study conducted in the Netherlands that included physical and mental tests among 5,000 people between the ages of 55 and 94 supports this theory. Researchers there found that those with artery disease, including plaque or heart attacks and strokes, had lower mental performance, no matter how old they were.

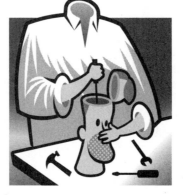

"If you want to continue to be sharp, if you want to continue to function effectively, then keep that blood pressure down," Dr. Elias says. "And if you can do that by natural means, by weight loss, by eating right, and by keeping that cholesterol down, it's going to pay off. You're going to be a sharper person, no question about it."

Are Antioxidants the Answer?

Any time you talk vascular health—even in the brain—the question is bound to come up: What role can the antioxidants beta-carotene and vitamins C and E play?

Like politicians staying on message, most medical experts advocate eating five to nine servings of fruits and vegetables a day to get the blood vessel–preserving effects of antioxidants. Frankly, they'd rather push carrots, cantaloupe, and sweet potatoes than supplements.

But either way, there's solid evidence that these dietary rustproofers seem to help preserve blood vessels and arteries by quenching free radicals—those hostile molecules that thrash around your body damaging cells. In the same way that soaking a slice of apple in orange juice—packed with vitamin C, we might add—prevents an apple from turning brown, antioxidants are thought to protect artery walls. This, scientists say, helps prevent low-density lipoprotein (LDL), the so-called bad, cholesterol from hardening the arteries and slowing blood flow.

Okay, you say, thanks for the remedial health education lesson. But how does this apply to brain function? Read on, Einstein.

Two big studies—the Nurses Health Study and the Massachusetts Elderly Cohort Study—seem to show the antioxidant beta-carotene kicking some serious nutritional butt—in this case by helping prevent stroke. Meanwhile, employees of a Swiss drug firm who didn't have as much beta-carotene in their blood were more likely to die from stroke. And, according to another study, supplementing beta-carotene cut the risk of "major vascular events"—no doubt, affecting brain function—by

---

Ginkgo Biloba: Chinese for "Smart"?

The name itself is enough to make you scratch your head. But if you're having trouble extracting those all-important bits of information from your mental recesses, you might want to consider taking ginkgo biloba extract (GBE).

Long used in the Far East and Europe, it's thought that this ancient herb helps boost blood flow to the brain and other parts of your body, says Dr. William J. Keller of Samford University.

Although more research needs to be done, chemicals in GBE may not only help open arteries and blood vessels but also, like vitamin E, help make blood less sticky.

Studies show that taking GBE can improve memory and mood, among other things. "Even older individuals, geriatric patients, seem to think more quickly and remember better when they take ginkgo," Dr. Keller says. "It's interesting stuff." It can be bought over the counter, and there have not been any problems associated with its use, even over the long term. The usual dose is 40-milligram tablets or capsules three times a day.

---

54 percent among doctors with chronic stable angina. Are we beginning to see a pattern here?

If not, here's more evidence courtesy of the guys in white lab coats.

- Another group of researchers waded into the information from the huge Netherlands study and said that the results seem to show that eating beta-carotene-rich foods helps protect against what they called cognitive impairment in the participants.
- Early findings from an offshoot of the Honolulu Heart Study indicate that

taking vitamin C and E supplements may protect the cognitive functioning of Japanese-American men.

- Mice given the equivalent of a human dose of 400 international units (IU) of vitamin E daily were found to have much less age-related damage to key parts of brain cells. This could lead to breakthroughs in treating such illnesses as Alzheimer's disease, suggests Marguerite Kay, M.D., professor of microbiology, immunology, and medicine at the University of Arizona College of Medicine in Tucson.

"There does seem to be some evidence that antioxidants reduce the risk for vascular disease and might help to maintain brain function," says Karen Riggs, Ph.D., research psychologist at the U.S. Department of Agriculture (USDA) Human Nutrition Research Center at Tufts University in Boston. "One of the ways good nutrition could help in maintenance of cognitive abilities is through staving off vascular diseases."

Until the results are carved in scientific granite, try to get at least the Daily Value of these nutrients.

The Daily Value for vitamin E is 30 IU, but most experts agree that you need 200 to 400 IU to get a protective effect—and it's hard to get that much without taking a supplement. Don't take more than 600 IU a day without consulting a health professional, says Vernon Mark, M.D., emeritus director of neurosurgery at Boston City Hospital.

Beta-carotene is a little trickier. Two large studies of long-term smokers have found that high daily doses of beta-carotene supplements—20 to 30 milligrams, or roughly four to six carrots—may up the risk of

Remember Your Lecithin

Don't go out and hijack a truckful of Ben and Jerry's, but there's evidence that a common ingredient added to foods like ice cream, mayonnaise, margarine, and chocolate bars can help preserve your memory.

Called lecithin, it's used by food manufacturers to help combine fat with water in some foods and as a natural antioxidant to prevent others from turning color. But lecithin also contains choline, a chemical that your body turns into acetylcholine, a neurotransmitter vital for brain function.

You probably can't get enough lecithin from these foods to make a big difference in your memory. But studies seem to show that taking lecithin or choline supplements, which are available in most health food stores, can help brain function.

During one study volunteers were divided into groups according to their ages: 35 to 50, 50 to 65, and 65 to 80. The groups were then subdivided, with half taking 3.5 grams of a form of lecithin a day and the other half taking placebos—fake pills. At the end of the three weeks, those who took the lecithin recorded almost half as many

developing lung cancer. Until we know more, it's probably best to stick with a beta-carotene supplement that contains no more than 6 milligrams, says Dr. Mark. Since your body converts beta-carotene into vitamin A when it is needed, some people elect to take vitamin A supplements. That is discouraged because fat-soluble vitamins, such as vitamin A, are retained in the body and may build up to toxic levels in the liver, Dr. Mark says. Go the food route. You will also get hundreds of other substances that may be beneficial to your health.

You can get the Daily Value of vitamin C—60 milligrams—from a single orange. So upping that with a supplement or by eating black

memory lapses on average—such as remembering names and retrieving misplaced items, according to Florence Safford, doctor of social work, associate professor of social work and gerontology at Florida International University in Miami and co-author of the study.

Perhaps most surprising, the folks between 35 and 50 had the greatest improvement. "Most of these were professionals, and a few of them told me that they were able to make speeches more extemporaneously—they found that they weren't searching for words as much. The improvement was really very dramatic," Dr. Safford says. "I use it and know it works. I just wish more people would try it for themselves. I recommend 1 to 2 tablespoons of lecithin granules. Some people may have gastrointestinal problems and should not take it, although I know some people who developed a tolerance for it by starting with a smaller dose of 1 teaspoon."

If you wanted to try to boost your intake naturally, eggs, beef, peanuts, and cauliflower are foods that are high in lecithin.

currants, red peppers, or strawberries should be a snap. Just remember, too much vitamin C will cause diarrhea in some people.

Putting the B in Brain

It's true that antioxidants are the stars of the vitamin world, high-profile players that you want to build your overall nutritional team around. But when it comes to keeping you eligible for that Mensa membership, some B vitamins are great role players. "For instance, a loss of vitamin B_1 (thiamin) produces neurological deficits, such as beriberi," says Dr. Mark. "Too low a level of vitamin B_{12} leads to other neurological deficits such as decreased reflexes and confusion. The question now, really, is how."

For years, researchers have talked about the link between B vitamins and neurotransmitters. The reason is simple: Several studies show that folks with higher levels of these B vitamins have better mental performance.

In one particular skull session, those folks between the ages of 54 and 81 with plenty of vitamin B_6 did well in what's called an activity memory test—a test that measures how well you can remember a sequence of things, like whether you cut the grass as the wife had asked before you watched basketball. And when it was time to see how well the same guys were able to copy increasingly complex shapes onto a paper—a skill admittedly not in great demand since about the time of the Dead Sea Scrolls—those with lower B_{12} levels did the worst.

In another study researchers found that taking 50 milligrams of thiamin a day for two weeks was found to increase mental retention time in adult males, compared to men who took a placebo—a fake pill.

And when researchers in the Netherlands added 20 milligrams of vitamin B_6 to the diets of healthy older men for three months, the guys' memories made significant gains, especially in long-term memory.

The Homocysteine Connection

As it turns out, B vitamins may do more than help build neurotransmitters and the sheaths that protect your nerves; they might actually help prevent brain damage. Researchers have discovered that when your body's supply of B_{12}, B_6, and folic acid are low, levels of an amino acid in your blood called homocysteine start to rise. And homocysteine, which has been linked to cardiovascular disease, may directly hinder the brain or cause mini-stroke-like conditions that decrease blood flow and brain function.

"It may be that one of the major ways that good nutrition affects cognitive function is through prevention of vascular disease. If so, then individuals would want to keep their homocysteine levels down. They would also want to keep their cholesterol within reasonable bounds. What you eat certainly affects those," says Dr. Riggs. "You should also make sure that there is some balance of B vitamins in your diet. Taking large doses of folic acid without enough B_{12} in your diet could put you at greater risk for problems associated with B_{12} deficiency."

Folate, the natural form of folic acid, is found in beans and green, leafy vegetables. The Daily Value for folic acid is 400 micrograms. Folic acid supplementation may only lower homocysteine levels effectively if there are adequate levels of vitamins B_{12} and B_6.

And don't forget riboflavin. This B vitamin helps folate and vitamin B_6 undergo the chemical transformation that allows them to do their thing.

Boring in on Boron

It doesn't even have a Daily Value. But some researchers say that boron—found in fruits and vegetables—can have a big impact on brain function.

During one study, 15 people were fed a low-boron diet—chicken, beef, pork, potatoes, rice, bread, and milk—for two months. The results weren't so swift, brain-wise: Eye-hand coordination, attention, perception encoding, and short-term and long-term memory all suffered at some point during the study. In fact, during electrophysiology tests (electroencephalogram tests measure brain electrical activity), the low-boron brains showed similar activity to those "often observed in response to general malnutrition and heavy metal toxicity," according to

Dr. James Penland of the USDA–Agricultural Research Service Grand Forks Human Nutrition Research Center.

"We also looked at actual cognitive performance with low intakes. So between the two measures, the cognitive measures and the measures with brain electrophysiology, it provides a pretty convincing case that lower intakes are not as good, not as healthy, for mental function as perhaps the slightly higher intakes are," says Dr. Penland.

To get these benefits, you need only boost your boron intake to between 1 and 3 milligrams a day. "You get a milligram from 1½ cups of applesauce, or 2½ cups of grape juice, or a little wine, or vegetables, such as broccoli. There is essentially none in animal products," explains Dr. Penland. "I know which ones I'd choose."

Zinc: The Thinking Man's Mineral

Metal is probably not the first word you associate with brainpower, especially if you've ever seen MTV.

But some researchers believe that there's a clear link between zinc and better thinking. In one study, researchers found that volunteers who took 10 milligrams of zinc a day—an amount that's actually less than the Daily Value, yet thought to be adequate—scored better on mental performance tests than those who took 4 milligrams or less.

"We actually saw an improvement in a variety of mental functions, including memory," says Dr. Penland. "And this helps confirm another study that found that women who took zinc sulfate supplements had improvement in nonverbal memory. It wasn't a fantastic improvement, but an improvement nonetheless."

Yet fewer men than ever may be getting the zinc they need to stay smart. Many guys are trying to trim fat from their diets by eating less beef. "They are denying themselves the richest sources of iron and zinc, and I'm not sure how wise that is," says Dr. Penland.

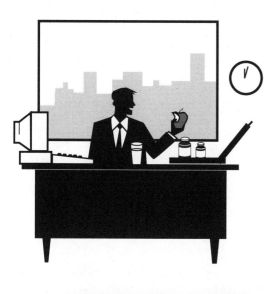

Part Six

Real-Life Scenarios

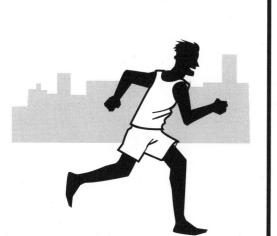

Quest for the Best

These men have worked hard to reach the top. And along the way, they have learned how vitamins and minerals can give them an important nutritional edge. Here are their secrets to success.

You Can Do It!

Just like you, these men struggle to find the time to eat right in these fast-paced times. To increase their odds of success, they have learned how to supplement smartly. So can you.

Quest for the Best

These men have worked hard to reach the top. And along the way, they have learned how vitamins and minerals can give them an important nutritional edge. Here are their secrets to success.

Bill Romanowski, Professional Football Player

Staying Strong on—And off— The Field

Bill Romanowski hasn't missed a day of work in 9 years. Not bad for a guy who toils in a profession where the average career lasts just 3½ years. Romanowski is a linebacker with the Denver Broncos. Now in his early thirties, he has never missed a game during an NFL career that has seen him star for the Super Bowl champion San Francisco 49ers and Philadelphia Eagles.

The six-foot-four, 241-pound Romanowski studies the latest nutrition reports as avidly as he does game films of upcoming opponents. He started to believe in the positive effects of eating well early on, as a high school football player in Rockville, Connecticut.

"I had a terrible diet until my sophomore year in high school," says Romanowski. "Then I read an article on Herschel Walker that said he did push-ups on his own and didn't eat fast food, so I started to eat a lot better. I would ask for apple juice when I went to a pizza place." His friends gave him a hard time, but Romanowski had his eye on a professional career and chose to model himself after a pro.

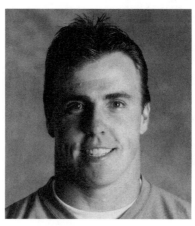

"The real change has come since I've been in the pros," Romanowski says. "Now, I can feel a difference if I don't eat properly or stop taking my nutritional and vitamin supplements."

Supplementing His Career

Like a lot of guys, Romanowski took supplements on and off over the years but could never get into a consistent habit. Then he consulted with his running coach Randy Huntington, who prompted him to have his blood and urine mineral levels tested by BALCO Laboratories in Burlingame, California.

"They told me that I was deficient in zinc, magnesium, chromium, and copper, which really surprised me because I consider myself to be a man who eats well and is very healthy," says Romanowski. "But when I talked to the people at BALCO Laboratories, they explained that a lot of the minor health problems I've had over the years were related to my deficiencies." For instance, Romanowski had always been a restless sleeper, and the director of BALCO Laboratories, Victor Conte, believed that this was due to his lack of magnesium.

"Sure enough, now I take magnesium before I go to bed every night and I sleep fine," Romanowski says.

Along with the magnesium, Romanowski's supplement regimen now includes zinc, chromium, a multivitamin with antioxidants and beta-carotene, and copper. "I learned that if I take the supplements all at once, some of the minerals will cancel each other out," he explains. "So I take them at specific times during the day." He takes a formula at night called ZMA that contains zinc and magnesium, chromium and copper 90 minutes before lunch, and his multivitamin/antioxidant with lunch.

To this mix of vitamins and minerals, Romanowski adds an advanced protein formulation called Proto Whey, which helps him add extra protein to his diet.

This kind of high-tech nutritional testing is common with Olympic athletes, says Romanowski, but is far rarer in professional sports. "My running coach trains Olympic athletes, and I see a lot more discipline in those guys," he says. "They think a lot more about what they eat and their other health habits."

Living Right Year-Round

Romanowski's view of good health looks like a triangle. There's a nutrition side, a recovery side, and a workload side.

"I basically eat a high-carbohydrate, low-saturated-fat diet with lots of chicken and fish about once a week," Romanowski says. "My total protein intake is 250 to 300 grams every day, which is why I supplement with Proto Whey."

He also drinks a half-gallon of water or more every day. "I always have water with me." Romanowski adds. "I've really noticed a difference since I got into that habit."

Just like his diet and workout, his recovery is also intense. Daily massages complement the 8 to 9 hours of sleep he gets every night.

"During the season I work out about 2 hours a day," Romanowski says. "I lift after practice three or four days a week." It's during the off-season, however, that Romanowski

really shows his dedication.

"I have to stay in absolute peak condition to keep my job. It's so competitive. I have to stay on top of things," Romanowski says. "I have my own running coach and massage therapist."

A third-round draft pick out of Boston College in 1988, Romanowski spent his first six seasons with the 49ers. He earned two Super Bowl rings and led the team in tackles four times before being traded to the Eagles in 1994.

It was during his two seasons with the Eagles that Romanowski started doing yoga, a discipline he practices as often as possible. In a move that would surprise many hardcore football fans, the Eagles had a yoga teacher on staff.

"I couldn't believe how much better I felt after I was doing yoga," says Romanowski. "I was doing it three times a day in training camp. The progress I made was incredible. I tried to keep it up on my own."

Football may be a glamorous job, but it's also a stressful one. Romanowski remembers reading once that professional football players have a life expectancy of 50 years. "That has probably changed, but reading that really had an effect on me. The old-timers didn't take care of their bodies, didn't work out properly, and didn't eat properly," he says. "I love what I do, but it's not worth it if I'm going to die at an early age."

Of course, football careers themselves end early in life, but despite the brutal hits that are part of his gridiron life, Romanowski believes that he takes good enough care of himself to live a long and healthy life.

"I have aging concerns just like anyone. I'm not only interested in helping my career," he says. "I want to knock out my chances of developing heart disease or cancer. I'm concerned about my overall well-being. No question.

"I'm always looking to improve my health. I read everything about nutrition that I can get my hands on," adds Romanowski. "My wife is even a nutrition major in college."

Pat Croce, Sports Franchise Owner

A Champ at Nutrition and Life

Philadelphia residents will have to forgive Pat Croce if their world-famous cheese steak isn't part of his regular diet.

It's not as if Croce lacks civic pride: Part owner of the NBA's Philadelphia 76ers and the NHL's Philadelphia Flyers, Croce once told a reporter that he'll have the members of his motorcycle "club" (called the Road Pirates) lead the parade when one of his teams brings a championship back to the City of Brotherly Love.

Nor is it because Croce doesn't enjoy that one-of-a-kind beef, onions, peppers, Cheese Whiz, pass-the-salt, make-sure-you-give-me-plenty-of-napkins-will-ya? taste.

It's just that Croce knows enough about nutrition to steer clear, except on special occasions. "If (NBA Commissioner) David Stern or (singer) Jimmy Buffet says, 'Let's go have a cheese steak,' I'll go have one," he says. "But it's a rarity. I have a complex about eating that much fat."

Such restraint is but one example of Croce's laserlike discipline. And once trained on a goal—whether it's eating right, winning an international karate competition, or owning a professional sports franchise—the question is not whether Croce will achieve it but when.

Always the Right Bite

Nutrition and healthy eating were an important part of Croce's life long before he took the helm of the 76ers. A licensed physical therapist and certified athletic trainer who built and sold a chain of physical therapy centers for $40 million, Croce was infamous for helping whip overweight professional athletes into shape. Among his many clients were a decidedly plump, nearly 300-pound Sir Charles Barkley, back when he was affectionately known as the Round Mound of Rebound.

It wasn't enough to make tough guys like Barkley puke from near exhaustion on their way to a sleeker frame. Croce believes that nutrition is at least a third of the equation. "Proper nutrition, proper training, and proper rest," says the sleek, six-foot, 165-pounder. "That's how it works."

His workouts literally come first. Before breakfast, Croce either runs 5 to 7 miles and does 60 pushups; performs a circuit aerobic/weight training program featuring upper-body and rowing ergometers, a StairMaster, and a Schwinn Airdyne bike; or does a 2-hour karate session.

He'll eat breakfast afterward, normally choosing either a whole-grain bagel covered with low-fat peanut butter and jelly (carbohydrates and protein); Frosted Mini-Wheats, raisins, and skim milk (carbohydrates and protein); or two large bran muffins (carbohydrates and fiber)—but always capped with a tall glass of orange juice, chock-full of vitamin C, and a multivitamin.

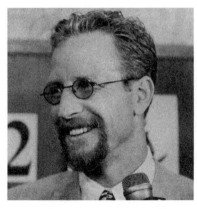

Croce shows his Philly roots at lunch by dining on pizza with peppers and mushrooms—even if he does ask the guys in the back to go easy on the cheese. Another favorite: Tuna on whole-wheat minus mayo. And then there's that great little deli—Norm and Lou's—by his office at the CoreStates Center where his team plays. "They have great turkey specials. Real turkey breast with a little coleslaw and light on the Russian dressing. As you can imagine, pretty low in fat," says Croce.

Mid-afternoon, Croce will top off his tank with a handful of pretzels. It's a healthy snack that he apparently shares with others. After one summer ride with his biker buddies, for example, Croce reportedly invited the gang over for pretzels and diet soda.

Half Italian, he prefers pasta for dinner, but even then he goes for the right bite. "Never fettuccine Alfredo or the cheese sauces. Always marinara," says Croce. More often than not, the pasta accompanies chicken or fish—broiled, of course.

His Way

You can bet that you'll never see Croce scarfing down a hot dog at a 76ers game. And not just because the boss gets special treatment. "They make me broiled crab cakes over penne pasta marinara. Or scallops over linguine. So if I get my protein with my carbohydrates and a salad, I'm fine," he says. You will see him drink a beer at the game. But wouldn't you know, it's a light.

Life on the road with the team can be tough, but more so when they aren't winning, he says. "No matter where you are, I think that you can always find healthy food," he says. "It's the game that we have to play when it comes to nutrition."

And those dinners for various celebrities and sports stars on the rubber chicken circuit? Croce doesn't hesitate to call ahead to see what's on the menu—or skip eating entirely if the meal is a nutritional disaster.

"Like last night. They had broccoli on the plate, which is good, and angel hair pasta, but it just had too much sauce on it. So you have to ask, 'Can I have this without the sauce?'"says Croce.

Does Croce's insistence on eating right mirror his success in the game of life? It may seem like an extreme example, but look no further than Croce's acquisition of the 76ers. "It

was the late 1980s during the playoffs when I said to the owner at the time, Harold Katz, 'If you ever plan to sell any part of the team, please give me a call.' And he laughed."

Croce never really stopped asking, finally cobbling a deal together with Comcast Cable, a Pennsylvania-based telecommunications company, to help bankroll the $125 million purchase of the team from Katz.

Or how about the way Croce returned to international karate competition after a 10-year hiatus, only to claim a gold medal at the age of 40—battling guys half his age. He might have won a gold medal the following year, too, but he was penalized for "excessive contact."

Persistence Personified

For such a competitive, hands-on guy like Croce, the 76ers' growing pains have been a real learning experience. "You can do everything right—from promotions, marketing, and sales to finance, management, and public relations—but you can't control the last 2 minutes of the game," he says. "You have to let it go. And boy, is that hard."

But Croce says that he intends to apply the same persistence and determination to the rebuilding of the once-mighty squad. A franchise that has counted two of basketball's true immortals—Julius "Dr. J." Erving and Wilt "The Stilt" Chamberlain—among its members. "I'm disciplining myself to be patient, if that makes any sense," he says. "Otherwise you would go nuts. It's going to take a while. There's a learning curve for everyone—from the general manager to the players and the coach. We have one of the youngest teams in league. It's brand-new. And you aren't going to be able to take it from the bowels of the league to the spotlight overnight...I want to. I'm trying to. But I can't get frustrated because it's not happening overnight. It's going to take discipline."

And Croce has no shortage of that.

Scott Connelly, M.D., Chairman and Founder of MET-Rx USA

Success He Can Shake On

For many years only one man benefited from the high-protein, high-nutrient shakes that now sell in health food stores across the country: their inventor, Dr. Scott Connelly. A cardiac anesthesiologist, he has measured, poked, and prodded his own body to test whether the line of supplements he concocted—MET-Rx—could keep him fit, trim, and energetic.

He considers himself the living proof.

A New Way

Dr. Connelly's quest for a fit body began when he became enamored with weight lifting during his teenage years in Texas. At the time his coach advised him to consume "protein and then more protein"—including 20 eggs, a gallon of milk, and 2 pounds of red meat every day. "Fortunately, I had a grandmother who loved to cook for me," he says. "I had a steak and 5 eggs for breakfast and then took hard-boiled eggs as well as meat sandwiches to school with me. I ate all day long just to get the food in."

An adolescent "hormonal milieu" combined with high-intensity weight training can handle this kind of caloric input, Dr. Connelly says, and feel great. "I was big and strong and felt like Hercules," he adds. His only supplementation at the time was a whole bunch of B vitamins.

Dr. Connelly's life changed suddenly and dramatically. "I had a traumatic injury to my leg with almost 3½ years of impaired mobility," he recalls. He lost huge amounts of muscle, dropping from 270 pounds to 130 pounds on a six-

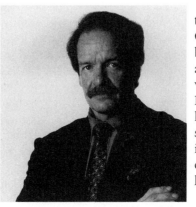

foot-five frame. Eventually, to mend his leg, Dr. Connelly took up walking and then jogging.

"Right about that time I got into medical school, and throughout my residency and fellowship I took up long-distance running as a way to get my body back into shape," Dr. Connelly says. "I also started to curtail my food intake to keep my body weight at a reasonable end point." His diet included a lot of pasta, like many serious endurance athletes. His weight steadied at about 160. Dr. Connelly first worked at Massachusetts General Hospital in Boston, then moved to Stanford University Hospital, where he was part of a faculty team in the intensive care unit (ICU).

"I saw immediately a correlation between me and the patients in ICU," Dr. Connelly says. "In the course of curtailing my food intake and running I didn't have a problem with weight, but my body composition was changing. Likewise, we were feeding patients thousands of calories, and yet they were wasting away."

Dr. Connelly began to challenge the prevailing idea that calories and calories alone make a person heavy. "I came to believe that to stay lean and strong you need to replicate some of the circumstances of growth," Dr. Connelly explains.

He turned to the agriculture industry for proof. "Our scientific community has far more data on how to manipulate the body composition of animals for meat production than how to manipulate a human being's body composition," he says.

At the end of the day two things can happen, says Dr. Connelly: Either your food can be burned up or it can be stored as fat or muscle. Carbohydrates will primarily be stored as fat, so Dr. Connelly, who had a long history of taking deliberate measurements of both his food intake and his body composition since his weight lifting days, changed his life.

"I stopped running and

went on a high-protein diet to complement my weight training program, which was designed to enlarge muscle mass," he says. His workouts comprised progressive intensity work, never using one muscle group more than once a week. He exercised for about 90 minutes, four times a week. "I was very fatigued at the end of each workout," Dr. Connelly says. "But I did muscle biopsies to chart the growth of fibers and found signs that I was on the right track."

Meanwhile, Dr. Connelly cut carbohydrates from about 60 to 70 percent of his diet to just 40 percent, filling the gap with lean protein. His total caloric intake increased from 2,500 calories a day to approximately 4,000 to 4,500 calories a day.

"The impact of that was enormous," Dr. Connelly says. "In a period of one year I gained 70 pounds of lean mass with just manipulation of diet and exercise. I experienced complete eradication of periods of low energy, and my mental acuity and my ability to persevere under an intense schedule markedly improved. "

Dr. Connelly's schedule looked like this: He would get up at about 5:00 A.M. and have "a protein concoction, which are now the shakes I sell commercially," he adds. Three to 4 hours later he would have a bran muffin or bagel, followed by another protein shake at lunch with some chicken breast or turkey. (He would grill or parboil a lot of meat on the weekends and take 8 to 10 ounces with him each day to work.) Another shake for an afternoon snack and then, yes, another shake for dinner, plus more chicken, turkey, or tuna. Sometimes he added a little carbohydrate or juice at the end of the day. "I don't like vegetables," he adds.

Dr. Connelly's diet hasn't changed much over the years. He still has six shakes a day. "My vitamin and mineral intake was always higher than most people's because the shakes are fortified with nutrients," he says.

MET-Rx follows the research closely, and Dr. Connelly is working on adding the nutritional "goodies," as he calls them, that have been shown to be beneficial. "I now take lycopene and luteine as well as six different

carotenoids," he says. "And I'm looking forward to taking a unique isoflavone. All these things will eventually make their way into MET-Rx." Dr. Connelly also takes saw palmetto as a preventive measure against prostate cancer.

Living Proof

So, what's missing from his regimen? Well, he doesn't feel the loss himself, but most other guys would.

"I have divorced myself from the typical thinking that regards food as a social or sensual event," says Dr. Connelly. "This is the one arena in which I am really at one extreme. Obviously, this isn't the average experience."

Interestingly, Dr. Connelly's most strident polemic is delivered against those couch-potatoes who scarf up loads of calories after dinner. "I can't overstate how deleterious it is to eat 60 percent of your calories in the evening," he says. "Calories should be spread throughout the day rather than eating them all in one sitting."

Dr. Connelly left the operating room at the end of 1993 to focus on the growth of MET-Rx, which was, he explains, "geometric." The change was extremely difficult for him. "I don't know bupke about running a company," he says. Under Dr. Connelly's direction, though, MET-Rx went from $300,000 in total sales in 1992 to $85 million in sales in 1996.

But more important, he is, once again, living proof of MET-Rx's success. "I'm in my late forties, and I look better than most 20-year-olds, which is a big kick for me," Dr. Connelly says. "I can't tell you with any accuracy whether I get fewer colds, but I can tell you that my cholesterol is going down, my blood pressure is low, and my resting pulse rate is about 48 beats per minute." Dr. Connelly claims only to have mastered the art of being fit; he hasn't found the secret to perfect health.

"MET-Rx represents the one opportunity I have to make a substantial and unique contribution to my field," says Dr. Connelly. "I started a revolution in an industry that once wallowed in fraud and voodoo."

Greg Isaacs, Trainer to the Stars

Building Bodies That Pass the Screen Test

He only has six months to help transform Kurt Russell into a buff-biceps action hero for an upcoming movie, but Greg Isaacs isn't worried.

"Kurt is a great athlete," says the creator and director of Warner Bros. fitness center in Burbank "He just has to get a little bit leaner and add some more muscle."

Motivating Russell doesn't seem to be a problem either. "He knows that he's the one who's going to be walking around in parts of the movie in a jockstrap, and that's motivation enough," says Isaacs. "I just remind him."

Isaacs has been down this road before. When supermodel/*Sports Illustrated* (SI) swim-suit vixen Vendela needed to add some pounds in all the right places before her first SI shoot—the folks at the magazine thought she was a little too skinny—Isaacs got the nod. Under Isaacs's tutelage, Vendela hit the weights, sprinted around the track, and ran the stairs at the University of California, Los Angeles (UCLA); ate right; and a few months later, was sporting more of those eye-catching curves. It sounds easy, but as Isaacs recalls, "She worked *hard.*"

In fact, some of the finest babes in Tinseltown, including Goldie Hawn and Melanie Griffith, have muscled up with Isaacs.

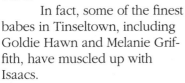

But, as he points out, even the hardest training and most genetically gifted among them wouldn't look nearly as good if they weren't eating right. "Let's face it, nutrition, eating right, is about 60 percent of the battle," Isaacs says.

Riding the Fitness Wave

Born in South Africa, Isaacs first began weight training at 13 when Arnold Schwarzenegger won a Mr. Olympia bodybuilding contest there. A trip a few years later to the land of endless bodies, Southern California, introduced him to the fledgling fitness movement.

After studying kinesiology and physical education, Isaacs returned to his homeland to open South Africa's first aerobics studio. He came back to Southern California as a personal trainer, hooking up with Johnny G., the inventor of the challenging, copyrighted bike workout known as Spinning.

When, at Clint Eastwood's suggestion, Warner Bros. decided to build a fitness center on the lot, Isaacs bested 10 competitors to win the contract to design, open, and manage the facility.

Since then, his list of clients—which already included tennis great Jimmy Connors, Don Johnson, John Lloyd, and Kathy Smith—expanded with a coterie of film industry executives. He has also written a book called *The Ultimate Lean Routine*, a 12-week cross-training and fat-loss program.

But unlike lots of books by "celebrities," their trainers, or both, Isaacs's no-nonsense approach is grounded in the idea that what you eat and when you eat it plays a critical role in shaping your physique.

Among Isaacs's many recommendations

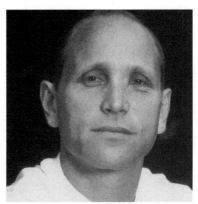

is eating 70 percent of your total calories before 3:00 P.M. and striving not to eat at all after 8:00 P.M. "I don't believe in letting yourself get hungry. I believe in keeping your blood sugar level as stable as you can."

Eating Right

Isaac's own nutritional program is guided by the number of killer workouts both he and his charges complete in a day.

Immediately after his morning 45-minute swim at the UCLA pool, Isaacs drinks water spiked with what may be the first legitimate superfuel in bodybuilding—creatine monohydrate—and vitamin C. But at five feet eight inches tall, 172 pounds, and a minuscule 6 to 8 percent body fat, Isaacs isn't using creatine to gain muscle.

"It's more to improve athletic performance because that's what I enjoy. There's nothing I like better than pounding out some miles on a bike, on the road, or in a pool," he says.

When he gets home, Isaacs will drink a shake made with one of the many whey-based protein supplements he uses, a banana, crushed ice, and apple juice. "I believe that you need to supplement your protein rather than taking it all in as meat. And besides, they almost always add vitamins and minerals to the protein powder," Isaacs says. (It's a good thing: Isaacs confesses that, like a lot of guys, he often forgets to take his multivitamin/mineral supplement). He may also eat a bowl of oatmeal and three or four egg whites.

A 45-minute run and light weight training with a client often follows. After that, he'll snack on yogurt or a banana. Then he's off to the next client for another weight workout or run.

By the time he gets to the Warner Bros. lot, it's lunchtime. And though the studio is known for creating films with some of the most sophisticated special effects around—the *Batman* series and *Space Jam* among them—the Warner Bros. commissary is straight out of an old-fashioned western: hot, heavy food and plenty of it.

As a result, Isaacs says that he'll bring a turkey sandwich topped with mustard, lettuce, and tomato or pasta with fresh tomato and tuna, plus chicken-and-rice soup, salad, and bread crusts from home to eat for lunch. For dessert, he'll nibble on a high-protein energy bar.

"It's a boring lunch, no question about it," says Isaacs. "And when I go to the cafeteria,

forget it. One day I had french fries and everyone goes, 'Uh-oh.' And then I say, 'You know, at least I can afford to eat french fries once in a while.' I eat pancakes, too. That's why I work out like a mother…so I can eat and enjoy. That's what this is about."

For dinner, Isaacs might have a small serving of pasta with turkey meatballs, or rice and steamed vegetables with chicken or fish, and a salad. And he expects his clients to eat the same way.

"I write out diets for them and give them to their cooks and their chefs. But that's part of the problem—you have to cook at your house. I said that to one of my clients. He went to the fridge and there wasn't anything to eat, and I said, 'You have to straighten your cook out.' You have to have protein with your pasta. You need to have some boiled eggs on hand. You have to have healthy snacks like yogurt and baked tortilla chips around so that you make wise food choices."

Other personal trainers may choose to rant and rave about such issues, but that's not Isaacs's style. "Don't get me wrong, I can be intense." he says. "But there's no need to scream. It's a matter-of-fact situation. Reality. I say, 'We have a job to do—let's do it.' There are young guys banging on the door that are trying to take your job."

And if that's not enough, Isaacs is constantly evaluating his clients' performance. "Every time I see them, I ask, 'What have you been doing? What did you eat yesterday? What's going on? Adjust, adjust, adjust.' That's what makes the difference.

"Anyone can learn the fundamentals of putting someone through a workout. Anyone can count reps. I try not to make small talk; I really try to focus in and concentrate. It's like, 'How are your abs feeling? Are we doing enough or not? Are you feeling fatigued?' It's not as if you have to do 25 and if you don't do 25, you're a piece of crap. Counting is insignificant. The question is, Do you feel it? Is your body changing? That's when you are successful."

You Can Do It! Just like you, these men struggle to find the time to eat right in these fast-paced times. To increase their odds of success, they have learned how to supplement smartly. So can you.

Ancient Wisdom, Modern Medicine

Ken Morris, Oakland, California

Date of birth: July 29, 1944

Height and weight: 5-foot-11, 156 pounds

Profession: Licensed acupuncturist, founder and director of the Institute for Chinese Herbology in Oakland, California

I grew up in Long Island, moved to California when I graduated from high school, and got married for the first time at age 19.

But during the late 1960s and early 1970s, I realized that the chaotic way in which I was living my life was no longer acceptable. I began then an investigation into the nature of my mind. I started to study tai chi and began to learn Chinese philosophy and medicine.

After two years in Burma and Southeast Asia studying the practice of meditation, I returned to the United States and became a licensed acupuncturist. A few years later I founded a school specializing in teaching Chinese herbal medicine.

Today I'm in my mid-fifties, and I consider myself in excellent health. I exercise every morning for about an hour around sunrise. My routine combines tai chi, yoga stretches, deep breathing, and some Pilates work, which combines stretching and calisthenics.

Afterward, I meditate for 45 minutes to an hour. I also do some form of aerobic exercise four times a week.

Although I was a vegetarian for more than eight years, I found that, working in an

urban environment, I needed a diet that made it easier to obtain high-quality protein. So I eat fish and organic chicken, and rarely pork, but never beef. I actually prefer to be a vegetarian, but I find that it takes a lot of time to do it properly.

When I started to use supplements I took the typical multivitamin. But then, as I learned more, I began to appreciate the complexity of taking a balanced intake of supplements.

Nutrition has a lot of variables to consider, and not all experts seem to agree on every issue. The good news is that these days there is a great deal of anecdotal and clinical information that supplements can enhance the quality of life.

Since then it has been a progression of experimentation. You have to learn to be sensitive to the changing needs of your body in order to determine what works for you. We need to be honest about how we really feel, not how we think we should be feeling.

These days I take a multivitamin/mineral supplement with 400 international units of vitamin E. Three times a day I take vitamin C supplements with other antioxidants.

My other supplements include DHEA (dehydroepiandrosterone) and coenzyme Q_{10} twice a day, various Chinese herbs, and other supplements as needed.

The cost of my regimen is $75 to $150 a month, depending on whether you pay wholesale or retail. Actually, I consider this amount a relatively inexpensive insurance policy.

Our bodies need continuing maintenance, especially as we age. While there is no preventing this degenerative process, we can learn to age more gracefully if we pay closer attention to our lifestyle.

On the Run, Staying Strong

Dan DeWitt, Brooksville, Florida

Date of birth: September 8, 1959

Height and weight: 6-foot-1, 195 pounds

Profession: Journalist

I've always considered myself a mediocre athlete. Not athletically gifted, but certainly someone who likes to stay fit. I started running when I was 12. I'd go out for occasional one-milers, which was four times around the park in front of our house. Of course, I never thought about vitamins and nutrition then. Who does at 12?

Later, in high school, I ran in the evenings with my father. He started running after his doctor told him that his unhealthy lifestyle was killing him. Later, I continued running in college, where I joined the cross-country team. For the most part, I've run on and off for most of the 16 years since. When injuries kept me from running, I rode a bicycle, played basketball (clumsily), and lifted weights instead.

For most of that time, I paid virtually no attention to my diet or other health habits. I started drinking in college, and if a fast-food restaurant was advertising a 99-cent sandwich, you can bet I'd be there.

When I started working for a newspaper, in my late twenties, I devoted most of my time to my job. As a reporter, I generally didn't sleep very well at night, partly because I kept myself wired on coffee throughout the day. As a result, I seemed susceptible to every illness that came around. I remember those years by what disease I got: A three-week bout with the flu during one year, bronchitis that wouldn't go away during another. I also remember that almost every Sunday I'd feel completely depleted after a long workweek and two days of partying.

The big change for me came about five years ago, when I was 32. I met my wife, Laura, who is a vegetarian and part-owner of a health food store and restaurant. Although many of my friends thought I was an incorrigible carnivore, Laura got me started on a meatless diet. (I did, and do, allow myself seafood, mostly at restaurants.) She also started me on a vitamin regimen. I began by taking two high-potency multivitamins a day. For me, this is a constant. I've sampled other supplements and found that DHEA (dehydroepiandrosterone) seems to help me build muscle. I also take glucosamine sulfate and shark cartilage connective tissue supplements as a way to battle periodic knee injuries. Like a lot of other people, I also take echinacea and additional vitamin C the moment I feel the hint of a cold coming on.

My overall impression of vitamins is that none of these supplements by themselves is an answer to better health. Although I'm sure they've done me some good, my habits have changed in so many ways that it's hard for me to determine the exact benefit. For example, a physical therapist showed me exercises for my knee injury, so is it the exercise or is it the joint supplements that now allow me to run further without pain? I'm not really sure. Do I get sick less often because of the echinacea and vitamin C or because I'm exercising more, eating a healthy diet, and trying to keep my stress down? Again, I'm not sure. But I do know that as long as I'm running better and not getting sick as often, I'm not about to drop the healthy lifestyle *or* the vitamins and supplements.

Although my life is more stable now, it's considerably busier. My wife and I have two young sons and an old house that requires a lot of maintenance. And my job certainly hasn't become any less demanding. But I'm more energetic now. In addition to not getting as sick as often, I find that I can concentrate better. And I have more patience. A lot of things have changed in my life. I'm not sure if the vitamins are the reason why I feel better, but I definitely think that they've contributed.

Growing Older, Feeling Younger

Bob Acquaviva, Tuckerton, New Jersey

Date of birth: July 8, 1948

Height and weight: 5-foot-8, 170 pounds

Profession: Self-employed in distribution

I grew up in South Philadelphia in a traditional Italian family. That means that all I ate was lots of pizza and spaghetti, plus pasta, cakes, and cookies. I hated vegetables and I never exercised. Somehow I managed to keep my weight steady at 170, but I certainly can't say that I was healthy.

In fact, I always had a lot of colds and viruses. I didn't think anything of it, and I never thought it was related to my diet. But I started to take vitamin C when I was in my late twenties and early thirties. It really helped tremendously. The colds subsided faster and the minute I went off the vitamins, I'd get sick.

Then, when I was about 40, I started to have really bad headaches and was always tired. I went to many different doctors to find out what was wrong. Finally, someone realized I had diabetes. Now, I've been living with this illness for almost eight years. I'm not insulin-dependent, but I am medicine-dependent.

When I found out about diabetes, my glucose levels were around 500. A nondiabetic has levels between 90 and 110. The doctor told me that if I didn't change my diet, I'd wind up on insulin.

I didn't start eating foods I don't like, but I did start eating more of the few vegetables I do like, such as spinach, corn, and beans. Unfortunately, I can't eat fruits that are high in sugar, like oranges or bananas, so that really limits my options.

I want to live a long time and I don't want to go on insulin, so I started to walk and lift weights. I could never even do one or two pushups; now I do 30 or 40 at a shot. Likewise, I bench-press 140 to 150 pounds when I lift weights. And I can walk miles and miles every day. Today, I feel about 15 years younger than I did when I first got sick.

Unfortunately, even though I felt better, I cheated a lot on my diet. I ate less pizza but still too much. So I started to need more medication. I was taking five pills in the morning, one in the afternoon, and another five at night. That's a lot of medication, especially for someone in his forties.

Then about eight months ago, I had a retina vein occlusion. That means that the retina ruptured and started to bleed into the nearby veins. I lost my sight in one eye, and the doctor said that there was no cure for it.

Now I've really started to change my habits, including doing some alternative nutritional therapy. I take a lot of vitamins and minerals, plus some herbs, that are designed to get the toxins out of my body. My nutritional doctor used to be a cardiovascular surgeon, but now he won't operate on people. Instead, he gives them high-dosage supplements.

Even though I went to this doctor out of desperation about my eye, the supplementation seems to be helping my diabetes. It has only been a few months, but I'm taking three fewer pills every day. My doctor is dropping the medication, but he won't attribute it to the vitamins or herbs or anything natural.

Aside from what this nutritional doctor gives me, I take vitamin C supplements two times a day. Plus, I take calcium and magnesium for the charley horses that I sometimes get while I sleep. Finally, I take chromium picolinate and a full-spectrum multivitamin/mineral tablet.

These days, my wife, Lorraine, and I eat more natural, unprocessed foods. I only eat pizza once every couple weeks. And I have to admit that I eat a lot of carrots for my eye.

Back home, they're still eating the way they used to, and they're always tired. Not me. Even with diabetes and my lost eyesight, I can work people under the table.

Banking on Health

Dave Gillan, Lewes, Delaware

Date of birth: April 3, 1960

Height and weight: 6 feet, 175 pounds

Profession: Bank officer

I'll be honest: I really don't find exercise and nutrition very exciting. In fact, I find working out and eating right boring, especially working out, which is hard for me to do unless I set myself specific goals. As for nutrition, I never gave it much thought when I was younger, and I follow it now mostly with a commonsense approach. I know and work out with plenty of guys who are fanatics with exercise, diet, and vitamins; but that's just not for me. The real reason why I try to stay healthy, work out, eat right, and take vitamins is simple: I want to be here when my kids are older. I want to be around when I'm 75, 80, 90 to see how they turn out. And how their kids turn out.

I started out like most people taking a chewable vitamin as a kid. I stopped by high school and didn't think much about vitamins or nutrition in college. Did you worry about nutrition in college? The only thing you worried about was the price of beer and making your first morning class on time. I never really noticed any problems from living like that in college, because one, I was young, and two, I was always active. (I played lacrosse and did martial arts.)

The real eye-opener was when I got my first job. It was in sales, and I was constantly on the road. My weight went up to something like 192, and it was all in my stomach. It was just embarrassing. When I moved back home, I opened a karate school and worked as a lifeguard during the day. When you're a lifeguard, you have to be in shape, and since I was competing a lot in karate tournaments, extra weight was a liability. I've been pretty good about staying in shape since then, including keeping a healthy diet, because it doesn't really make sense to put so much effort into exercise if you're going to fight against yourself by eating junk. I also keep on top of things now, I think, because I set specific goals for myself to stay in shape. One year it was triathlons, and I did about a half-dozen. My weight then was around 168, but I think that I was a little obsessed. Another goal was to swim 4½ miles in the Chesapeake Bay, which I did in June 1996. Another was to learn how to do jumps with my Windsurfer.

I really began to pay attention to vitamins a few years ago when they started getting really popular and when I was in my obsessive triathlon training. I remember reading how certain vitamins, like the antioxidants, are good for you. But I remember one doctor saying that you should get everything you need from your food and that people who pop 20 pills a day wind up with nothing but expensive pee.

That intrigued me, so I read a lot and talked to some nutritionists and my workout buddies about it. I decided that I wanted to take a good, healthy one-a-day multivitamin but that I wanted to get a little extra of the things I wanted, like antioxidants. Now I take a mega multivitamin from GNC. It costs about $20 for 90 tablets and has all that I'm looking for and then some. It has vitamins A, C, E, and D; thiamin; and riboflavin. I also take chromium picolinate when I'm training. It's supposed to burn fat and preserve lean muscle. I don't know if it really burns fat or preserves muscle, but I can tell you that my legs and body don't hurt as much as they used to at the end of the season.

The best thing now is that I enjoy being healthy with my whole family. My wife, Christine, takes vitamins; and my kids Grant and Taylor take chewables suggested by our doctor. My wife, who used to teach aerobics, does the stationary bike. She'll get up at 5:00 A.M. to ride. That's discipline that I can respect. The vitamins, the diet, and the exercise for us are a means to an end. Hopefully, they'll let me stay around a little longer and be a little healthier than I would without.

Index

Underscored page references indicate boxed text and tables. Boldface page references indicate primary discussions of topic.